T0220363

The Basics of Cancer Immunotherapy

Haidong Dong • Svetomir N. Markovic

Editors

The Basics of Cancer Immunotherapy

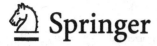

Editors
Haidong Dong
Department of Urology,
Department of Immunology
College of Medicine, Mayo Clinic
Rochester, MN, USA

Svetomir N. Markovic
Department of Oncology, Department
of Medicine/Division of Hematology,
Department of Immunology
College of Medicine, Mayo Clinic
Rochester, MN, USA

ISBN 978-3-319-70621-4   ISBN 978-3-319-70622-1   (eBook)
https://doi.org/10.1007/978-3-319-70622-1

Library of Congress Control Number: 2017961878

© Springer International Publishing AG 2018
This work is subject to copyright. All rights are reserved by the Publisher, whether the whole or part of the material is concerned, specifically the rights of translation, reprinting, reuse of illustrations, recitation, broadcasting, reproduction on microfilms or in any other physical way, and transmission or information storage and retrieval, electronic adaptation, computer software, or by similar or dissimilar methodology now known or hereafter developed.
The use of general descriptive names, registered names, trademarks, service marks, etc. in this publication does not imply, even in the absence of a specific statement, that such names are exempt from the relevant protective laws and regulations and therefore free for general use.
The publisher, the authors and the editors are safe to assume that the advice and information in this book are believed to be true and accurate at the date of publication. Neither the publisher nor the authors or the editors give a warranty, express or implied, with respect to the material contained herein or for any errors or omissions that may have been made. The publisher remains neutral with regard to jurisdictional claims in published maps and institutional affiliations.

Printed on acid-free paper

This Springer imprint is published by Springer Nature
The registered company is Springer International Publishing AG
The registered company address is: Gewerbestrasse 11, 6330 Cham, Switzerland

Acknowledgements

We are grateful to the pioneers, our mentors, and colleagues in the field of cancer immunology and immunotherapy. We dedicate our book to our patients and their families for fighting cancer with us. Our research has been supported by the National Institute of Health, the National Cancer Institute, and the Mayo Foundation. We appreciate Dr. Khalid Jazieh, MBBS, for helpful review of the drafts of each chapter and in designing several graphs and suggesting the idea for the cover design. We apologize for not being able to cite all of the excellent studies and clinical trials in this field due to space limitations.

Haidong Dong
Svetomir N. Markovic

Contents

Chapter 1
The Basic Concepts in Cancer Immunology and Immunotherapy

Haidong Dong

Contents

Why Do We Have Cancer?

Cancer is a cellular disease resulting from the uncontrolled growth of tumor cells. A massive amount of tumor cells accumulate in one or more parts of the body or spread throughout the blood. Documentation of human cancer can be found in literature dating as far back as 3,000 years ago in Egypt, and the search for the cause

H. Dong (✉)
Department of Urology, Department of Immunology, College of Medicine, Mayo Clinic, Rochester, MN, USA

© Springer International Publishing AG 2018
H. Dong, S.N. Markovic (eds.), *The Basics of Cancer Immunotherapy*,
https://doi.org/10.1007/978-3-319-70622-1_1

never comes to an end. While inheritance and environmental factors (ultraviolet radiation, pollution, etc.) are attributed as major causes of human cancer, a recent report pointed out that random errors in replication of genetic materials (genome) in our bodies seem to play a key role in cancer generation (Tomasetti et al. 2017). Once a genomic error happens, its consequence may or may not be harmful to our bodies and the cells harboring the error. The error or mutation (changes) in the genome can cause a normal cell to become a tumor cell. These errors in the genome are responsible for two-thirds of the mutations in human cancers (Greenman et al. 2007). In its early stages, a cancer cell does not look so different from other normal cells, yet they may behave differently, such as continuing to proliferate (divide) and consuming extra nutrients (higher metabolism). Contrary to normal cells, cancer cells have lost control over their proliferation; nothing can stop them until they take over the whole body. Since the errors that happen in our genome are random, most of our cancers may not be predictable or realistically preventable at the genetic level. However, not all mutations or errors in our cells will lead to cancer. We have both internal- and external-checking systems to monitor what happens to the cells in our bodies. If all these checking systems fail, tumor cells will proliferate and take control—the disease spreads throughout the body, eventually resulting in death if not treated.

The internal-checking system consists mainly of tumor suppressor genes that suppress the development and growth of mutant cells in a process called "pro-grammed cell death." In this process, some enzymes will be activated to cut the genetic material of cells into small fragments that will stop the proliferation and survival of the cells. Basically, our cells are programmed to die if they detect any mutations within their genes that they cannot correct. If the tumor cells escape this internal check, they will face an external check that is mediated by the immune system. Our immune system has developed the ability to check for tiny changes in cells. Immune cells have very specific "eyes" to identify any subtle changes in nearby cells. The "eyes" of immune cells are receptors that function to detect very specific changes in our cells and will activate our immune cells accordingly. Usually, these changes are in the proteins (structure and function molecules) expressed by tumor cells. Cancer cells usually harbor many altered and abnormal proteins due to errors in the genome coding the proteins, or due to uncontrolled production of some proteins that should have been shut down when cells matured past their early stages. Certain environmental factors may also cause damage in the genome that results in the production of altered proteins. When our immune cells detect these altered proteins on the surfaces of the tumor cells, they will recognize them, become activated, and eventually destroy the tumor cells. As long as our immune system can recognize these changes inside any cancer cells, the cancer cells cannot accumulate and develop into a disease. Therefore, cancer is ultimately a disease caused by unlimited growth of tumor cells that escaped the attack of the immune system.

How Does the Immune System Protect Us from Cancer?

Many of us have tumor cells in our bodies, but most of us do not develop cancer as a disease. Our immune system prevents spontaneously generated tumor cells from developing into cancers. This phenomenon has been reproduced in animal models and has prompted a theory of "immune surveillance." There are four pieces of evidence that support this theory that the immune system indeed responds to cancer. First, humans with genetic defects in their immune systems tend to have a higher incidence of cancer than those whose immune systems are intact. Second, humans who have their immune systems suppressed by medicine in order to avoid rejection of transplants have higher cancer generation than people with normal immune function. Third, some cancer patients have "paraneoplastic syndromes" that are caused by the immune system's response to a cancer. For example, patients with lung cancer may develop disorders in the central nervous system (CNS) due to immune responses to certain proteins shared by CNS and lung cancers. It is further proof that internal immune responses to tumors are present as they can even begin to attack the normal tissues that share the same proteins with tumors. Last but not least, immunotherapy has been used to treat some human cancers in recent years. Immunotherapy regimens do not directly kill tumor cells but boost the immune system to find and destroy cancer cells. The success of this therapy provides direct evidence that we have pre-existing immune responses to cancer in our body, but at times they do not function as well as they should. However, once we give them a boost, they will do a great job in attacking cancer.

Two Types of Immune Responses

The two types of immune responses differ in their specificity of recognition and speed of response. One is called the innate immune response, in which innate immune cells lack precise specificity in recognition of their targets but have a rapid response to them. Macrophages (large eater cells) and natural killer (NK) cells are the main innate immune cells. They recognize their targets based on the general patterns of molecules expressed by target cells or pathogens.

The second response is called the adaptive immune response. Adaptive immune cells have a very restricted specificity in recognition of their targets, but usually have a delayed response to their targets because they need more time to divide and produce attacking molecules. There are two major sub-populations of adaptive immune cells: T cells and B cells, also called T lymphocytes and B lymphocytes (since they were originally identified in lymph nodes). The "T" in T cells means that these cells develop in the thymus, and the "B" in B cells means they develop in bone marrow. They recognize their target cells or pathogens using receptors (eyes) that are designed only for a very specific antigen. An antigen is a protein molecule or any substance capable of inducing an immune response that produces antibodies (antigen-binding proteins) or attacking molecules. As this specificity is so detailed, T cells or B cells can recognize any tiny changes in a protein molecule. In order to recognize any potentially changed proteins or pathogens, our bodies have been bestowed with 300 billion T cells and 3 billion B cells. Normally we only have a few T cells for each single antigen in our bodies, but we can have thousands of them once they are activated by antigen stimulation and undergo expansion (proliferation). Although we cannot see the expansion of T cells, we can feel them. When you feel enlarged lymph nodes in your body after infection, these signs usually tell you that millions of immune cells proliferated.

Innate Immunity to Cancer

As we learned above, the innate immune response is fast, but not restricted to specific antigens. It is still unclear how innate immune cells recognize tumor cells, but they do have the ability to kill tumor cells once they are activated by environmental cues. Macrophages and NK cells are the two major types of innate immune cells that can attack tumors. There are other innate immune cells that do not directly kill tumor cells, but can present proteins expressed by tumor cells to other immune cells to instruct them to target these tumors. For example, dendritic cells (DCs) are innate immune cells that can present tumor proteins to adaptive immune cells (like T cells) and help activate T-cell responses; thus, the dendritic cells act as a "bridge" between the innate immune system and the adaptive immune.

Macrophages are big eater cells. Macrophages are present within most tissues of our body in order to clean up dead cells and pathogens. Once activated by environmental cues (like materials released from bacteria, viruses, or dead cells), macrophages infiltrate deep into tumor tissues and destroy cells via production of toxic oxygen derivatives (reactive O_2 intermediates) and tumor necrosis factor (TNF), or they directly eat the tumor cells (known as phagocytosis). In order to escape being eaten by macrophages, some tumor cells express "don't eat me" signal molecules to fool macrophages and escape them. Recently, reagents have been developed to block the "don't eat me" molecules on tumor cells. An example of a "don't eat me" molecule is CD47. CD47 on tumor cells interacts with signal-regulatory protein alpha (SIRP-α), an inhibitory receptor present on macrophages. Since engagement of CD47 with SIRP-α inhibits macrophage phagocytosis, blocking CD47 may enhance the "eating" of tumor cells by macrophages (Tseng et al. 2013). Thus, macrophages are "tumor" eater cells, but tumor cells can find a way to escape them. Recently, some drugs (e.g., CD47 antibody) that can help macrophages to eat tumor cells have been tested in clinical trials.

NK cells are circulating immune cells in our blood system and are believed to serve as the earliest defense against blood-borne metastatic tumor cells. In order for tumor cells to be recognized by NK cells, there must be something that distinguishes them from normal cells—such as expressing something abnormal and/or failing to express something normal. NK cells are called natural killers because they do not need to be "coached" to see very specific antigens for their activation. They respond to their target cells by searching whether something is "missing" on the cell surface. In this regard, NK cells help us clean out many cancer cells in very early stages or those cancer cells circulating in our blood where we have plenty of NK cells. Patients with metastases have abnormal NK activity, and low NK levels are predictive of eventual metastasis. Recent studies suggest that some NK cells have a "memory" capability to recognize certain tumors or pathogens. However, there are limitations in NK cell-mediated antitumor immunity. First, only tumor cells with "missing" markers can be detected by NK cells. Second, there are a limited number of NK cells present in the bloodstream, as only 10% of lymphocytes are NK cells. In addition, tumor cells can avoid NK cell attacks by expressing immune suppressive molecules to inhibit NK cell function, in a manner similar to how they can avoid getting eaten by macrophages. To improve NK cell function, a cytokine called interleukine-2 has been used to activate NK cells for expansion.

Adaptive Immunity to Cancer

In contrast to innate immunity, the adaptive response is slower, specific to certain antigens, and has memory (can provide life-long protection). Since adaptive immune cells can remember antigens from their first encounter, they can respond to antigens much faster when they encounter the same antigens again. This process is called "immune memory" and is the foundation of protective immunization. The eyes of adaptive immune cells are "near sighted." They need a very close cell-to-cell contact to clearly and specifically "see" their antigen on the target cells. In order to remember their target antigens, adaptive immune cells need professional antigen-presenting cells (APCs) to "teach" them how to see and how to respond. Dendritic cells are professional APCs. Dendritic cells are called "dendritic" because they have dendrites (branches) that extend to surrounding tissues to catch proteins released from pathogens or tumors, but they cannot eat whole cells like macrophages. Once they catch proteins (antigens), they will "eat" (phagocytosis) and "digest" them using enzymes (degradation), and then "present" them in an antigen-presenting structure on their surfaces. The antigen-presenting structure is called the major histocompatibility complex (MHC) that is a set of cell surface protein complexes that contain a "pocket" in order to hold an antigen. The main function of MHC is to display antigens on the cell surface for recognition by the appropriate T cells (Fig. 1.1). Thus, the MHC is like a gauge indicating whether there are tumor antigens within a cell to which the immune response will be turned on to them.

There are two types of adaptive immunity: cellular (T-cell) and humoral (B-cell) immunity. T cells consist of CD8 and CD4 T cells. CD8 T cells are also called cytotoxic T lymphocytes (CTLs). They are the primary killers of tumor cells because they can distinguish cancer cells from normal cellsand directly destroy cancer cells.

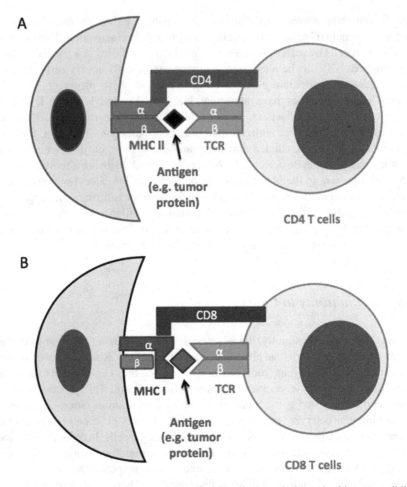

Fig. 1.1 Tumor antigen can be presented to CD4 T cells through the major histocompatibility complex II (MHC II) or to CD8 T cells through MHC I in order to activate T-cell receptors (TCRs)

CTLs kill cancer cells via a quick yet well controlled cell-to-cell contact process. They start by digging a hole in the cancer cells and inject enzymes that can dissolve their inner materials. Some injected enzymes can cut the genetic materials into very small pieces leaving the cancer cells to die in a manner known as apoptosis (a Greek word meaning falling apart). As for CD4 T cells, their major function is producing soluble proteins called cytokines. These cytokines are messages sent by CD4 T cells to regulate or help the function of other immune cells during an immune response. Some cytokines are called interleukins (ILs), because they deliver messages between leukocytes (white blood cells). CD4 T cells that use these messages to help other immune cells are called T helper cells (Th). We have several types of T helper cells according to their different production of cytokines (Th1, Th2, Th17, etc.). Among them, Th1 cells play a key role in suppressing tumor growth because they produce a cytokine called interferon (IFN)-gamma that can inhibit the growth of tumor cells. Some CD4 T cells also have a cytotoxic function like CTLs in killing of tumor cells.

In order to kill tumor cells but not normal cells, T cells need to specifically distinguish tumor cells from normal cells. They can do this because tumor cells, unlike normal cells, express unique tumor antigens that can induce T-cell responses. It took a long time for people to discover tumor antigens because they are embedded in MHCs, rather than standing alone on the cell surface as people originally perceived. Dr. Boon and his colleagues discovered the first human cancer antigen in melanoma (van der Bruggen et al. 1991). They found a way to "flush out" the small protein fragments (called peptides) that are embedded in a pocket of MHC. There are two classes of MHCs: class I and class II. The class I MHCs present antigens to CD8 T cells, and the class II MHCs present antigens to CD4 T cells. Class I MHC molecules are expressed by almost every cell in humans, while class II MHC molecules are restricted to certain immune cells like macrophages and lymphocytes. The antigen peptides presented in MHC are recognized by T-cell receptors (TCRs) expressed by T cells. TCR is very specific for each tumor antigen peptide in a particular MHC. A T cell only expresses one type of TCR and can only recognize one type of antigen.

Unlike T cells, B cells do not kill tumor cells directly, but produce antibodies as their attack molecules. Their antibodies function like "catchers" that can grasp their target antigens. There are five classes of antibodies: IgG, IgM, IgA, IgD, and IgE, based on their different chemical structures and functions. IgG is the major antibody type that crosses the placenta to provide protection for the baby. IgM is the largest antibody in our bodies. IgA can be released to our intestines to control infections in our digestion system. IgE is the major antibody to control parasites but also causes allergies. IgD functions like a receptor for the activation of B cells. Each antibody can only bind to one antigen. Once antibodies bind to antigens, they either block the function of their target molecules or direct other immune cells (like macrophages and NK cells) to kill the target cells that express the antigens, a process called antibody-dependent cell-mediated cytotoxicity (ADCC). ADCC plays a key role in the treatment of human cancers, especially cancer cells in the blood.

The Efficiency of the Immune System: The Power of Diversity

Since an immune (T or B) cell only can recognize a tiny part of an antigen and only a few cells have this specificity, the efficiency of the immune system in responses to any altered proteins or pathogens can be very low. To increase efficiency but not compromise specificity, diversity is granted to the immune system. This diversity is achieved at the genetic level in order to produce a battery of different kinds of receptors or antibodies for recognizing different antigens, and different MHC for presenting different antigens. Based on the gene arrangements that generate the diversity of MHC in a single cell, one cell can express at least 12 different MHCs that present at least 12 kinds of different epitopes of an antigen. An epitope is the smallest portion of an antigen protein that can be recorgnized by T cells. For example, if a pathogen virus infected a host cell, this host cell can present 12 kinds of epitopes of a viral protein. Accordingly, there will be at least 12 kinds of T cells that express receptors for each antigen epitope and will be able to recognize the viral antigens of the infected cells and destroy them in order to stop infection. In the case of tumor cells, if a tumor cell has two tumor antigens, the tumor cell can present at least 24 kinds of epitopes and will stimulate 24 kinds of T cells. Since only one T cell is enough to kill one tumor cell, if we have 12 or 24 kinds of T cells in place, we will have more than enough T cells to kill the tumor cells. Therefore, the diversity of our immune system is a crucial mechanism in protection and elegantly balances the specificity of each immune cell.

Why Does the Immune System Fail to Control Cancer Cells?

If the immune system has the ability to protect us from cancer, why do some of us develop cancer as a disease? It has been observed that in many patients, cancer cells are surrounded by immune cells in tissues or co-exist with tumor-reactive immune cells in the peripheral blood. Despite this, their cancer continues to progress and spread all over the body. We have a name for this enigma: the Hellström paradox, after Ingegerd and Karl Erik Hellström, two immunologists who first described this paradox more than 50 years ago (Hellström et al. 1968). In the last few decades, many efforts have been made to tip the balance in favor of the immune system based on the assumption that there are not enough immune cells to keep the cancer cells in bay. Most recently, we realized that even if there are plenty of immune cells capable of killing cancer cells, these immune cells can be killed or suppressed by cancer cells at tumor sites. The fight back from cancer cells is so powerful that many tumor vaccine therapies and T-cell transfer therapies failed to control cancer due to the barriers built up in the tumor sites. The discovery of B7-H1 (also named PD-L1) expressed by human tumor cells opened a door for us in our understanding of how tumor cells escape immune surveillance (Dong et al. 2002). PD-L1/B7-H1 is used by cancer cells to disarm the immune system and blocking of PD-L1 restores the antitumor function of immune cells (Dong and Chen 2003; Iwai et al. 2002). PD-L1 and other immune regulatory molecules (CTLA-4, PD-1, B7-DC/PD-L2, etc.) are collectively called "immune checkpoint molecules" as they function as barriers for restraining immune responses. Accordingly, immune checkpoint blockade therapy is applied to restore the function of tumor-reactive immune cells by lifting the checkpoint barriers (Pardoll 2012; Korman et al. 2006). The success of immune checkpoint blockade therapy also tells us that the suppression put on the immune system is reversible as long as we have the right tool to do so. In the following sections, you will learn how the immune system is regulated, how cancer cells usurp the self-protection mechanism for their own safety from immune cells, and novel strategies in the treatment of cancer based on new discoveries.

The Checks and Balances on the Immune System

While the diversity of our immune system protects us from pathogen infections or cancer cells, it also mounts a great risk for us to be attacked by our own immune system if this system goes out of control and responds to any changes identified in our bodies. To avoid the overreaction of our immune system, a battery of checkpoint molecules is put in place to check and balance our immune responses.

Immune cell activation means a status of immune cells where they proliferate more and produce molecules that affect the fate of targeted cells. However, it is not an easy job to activate immune cells. Only specific antigens trigger the receptors of immune cells, and these specific antigens function like a specific key that is used to turn on the engine of a car. Antigen stimulation alone usually is not able to activate T cells, just like a car cannot move faster when only the engine is turned on. To have the car move faster, we need to press down the accelerator pedal in order to inject more gasoline into the engine. The accelerators of immune cells are called co-stimulatory signals. Immune cells need co-stimulatory signals to become fully activated. For safety, we also need a brake system to control the speed or movement of a car. The brake system on immune cells is called immune checkpoint molecules. When we are driving a car, we frequently use both the gas pedal and the foot brake to balance the speed according to surrounding situations in order to have a smooth and safe drive to our destination. During a process of immune responses, immune cells also need to consistently receive both co-stimulatory and checkpoint signals in order to work specifically and efficiently in places where they are eliminating infected cells or cancer cells.

Mechanisms Used by Tumor Cells to Escape Immune Attack

First of all, cancer cells do their best to hide from the detection of the immune system. Since tumor antigens presented by MHC can reveal their identity to the immune system, most of the time, tumor cells turn down or even turn off their presentation of tumor antigens by downregulation of MHC (antigen-presenting complex) expression or production of tumor antigens. Tumor cells accumulate many mutations in their MHC molecules that prevent them from being appropriately expressed, thus dampening the ability of MHC to present tumor antigens. In addition to MHC, tumor cells may also turn off the machines that can produce tumor antigens inside cells.

Tumor cells also take the advantage of the brakes in the immune system. Tumor cells express immune checkpoint molecules to actively turn down the immune responses against them. One important molecule is called B7-H1, which was discovered at Mayo Clinic in 1998 (Dong et al. 1999). B7-H1 was renamed PD-L1 in 2000 because it was found to be a ligand (binder) of PD-1 (Freeman et al. 2000). PD-1 is another important molecule of the immune system that was discovered in

1992 (Ishida et al. 1992). PD-L1 is expressed by most human solid cancer cells (Dong et al. 2002). When activated immune cells that express PD-1 come to tumor sites and get closer to tumor cells, their PD-1 will be engaged by the PD-L1 expressed by tumor cells. Once engaged, PD-1 transmits signals into those immune cells that will cause them to either die or lose their immune function (Dong et al. 2002; Iwai et al. 2002). That is where PD-1 gets its name from—programmed death-1 molecule.

Therefore, it is no surprise that high expression of PD-L1 predicts poor survivorship of patients with renal cell carcinoma, lung cancer, ovarian cancers, and some other cancers (Thompson et al. 2006). By extension, therapeutically targeting the interaction of PD-1 and PD-L1 using antibodies that block this contact will be able to restore the antitumor function of immune cells. Recently, the US Food and Drug Administration (FDA) approved two anti-PD-1 drugs and three anti-PD-L1 drugs in the treatment of several human cancers. Of note, all these drugs are antibodies specific for PD-1 or PD-L1. Once these antibodies are injected into the blood of cancer patients, they will find their target molecules PD-1 on T cells or PD-L1 on tumor cells and bind to them. Once these molecules are bound by appropriate antibodies, the interaction of PD-1 and PD-L1 will be blocked, and tumor cells cannot use PD-L1 to engage PD-1 and suppress T cells that are capable of killing them (Fig. 1.2).

Before immune cells travel to tumor sites, their function is also regulated at lymph nodes that are close to tumor sites. Another immune checkpoint molecule called CTLA-4 (cytotoxic T lymphocyte antigen-4) is expressed by activated T cells. CTLA-4 provides negative feedback signals for T-cell activation. To release the regulation of immune cells at lymph nodes and promote their potential antitumor function, CTLA-4 blocking antibodies became the first regimen in cancer immune checkpoint blockade therapy (Leach et al. 1996). CTLA-4 not only regulates tumor-reactive immune cells, but also self-reactive immune cells in the lymph nodes. Thus, a global blockade of CTLA-4 has the risk in increasing autoimmune responses, some of which could be fatal. Caution should be exercised in monitoring patient responses to immune checkpoint blockade therapy, either PD-1/PD-L1 or CTLA-4, to avoid and prevent potential risks of autoimmune responses, which are called self-toxic effects.

In addition to these immune checkpoint molecules, tumor cells invite their "friends" to help them escape immune attacks. They attract myeloid-derived suppressor cells (MDSCs) to help them turn down the activation of immune cells within tumor sites or lymph nodes near the tumor tissues. MDSCs are bone marrow cells in the process of becoming antigen-presenting cells, but their normal development process is disrupted by tumor cells that recruit them to suppress antitumor immunity (Bunt et al. 2006). Lymph nodes and tumor sites contain another type of immune cells called regulatory T cells (Treg), which also help tumors by dampening immune responses (Curiel et al. 2004; Casares et al. 2003). Treg cells have the ability to inhibit the antitumor function of tumor-reactive immune cells by competing for their nutrition or reducing T-cell activation.

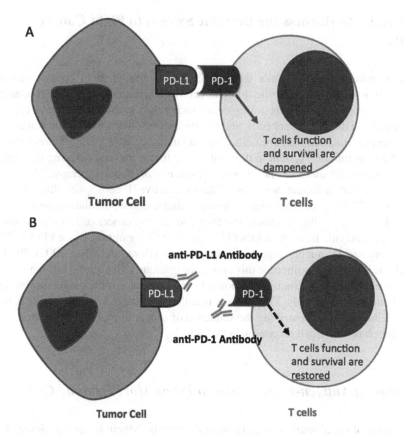

Fig. 1.2 (**a**) Tumor cells that express programmed death ligand 1 (PD-L1) activate the programmed death receptor 1 (PD-1) to inhibit T-cell function and cause T cells to die. (**b**) Antibodies that target PD-L1 or PD-1 can be used to stop tumor cells from suppressing T cells, allowing T cells to be reactivated to fight the cancer

Tumor cells can actively release soluble molecules to create an environment that is harsh to immune cells. They produce VEGF (vascular endothelial growth factor) not only to promote blood supply for themselves, but also to suppress the function of antigen-presenting cells (dendritic cells) and avoid having their identity exposed to the immune system. They also release cytokines (TGF-beta, IL-10, etc.) that directly inhibit the activation or function of immune cells. As we know, immune cells require a significant amount of energy to do their job, and to interfere with this an enzyme called indoleamine 2,3-dioxygenase (IDO) is produced in tumor tissues. This enzyme helps tumor cells use most of the essential amino acid tryptophan in the tumor environments, thus dramatically reducing the levels of tryptophan, which is a critical "food" for immune cells. When immune cells are starved of tryptophan, they lose their ability to fight cancer cells. To prevent that happening, drugs that block the function of IDO have been tested as cancer immunotherapy agents (Friberg et al. 2002).

Strategies to Harness the Immune System to Fight Cancer Cells

Cancer immunotherapy works through the immune system to control cancer; therefore, its direct target is the immune cells rather than the tumor cells. Cancer immunotherapy is aimed at restoring or enhancing the capability of immune cells to recognize and destroy cancer cells, and the therapeutic effects will be determined by the extent to which the immune cells eliminate tumor cells. While it is unreasonable to expect the immune system to deal with large tumor masses, reducing the tumor burden seems to increase the chance of success of immunotherapy. The ideal scenario is that sufficient numbers of tumor-reactive T cells (with "highly avid recognition") are generated by appropriate tumor-antigen stimulation, and T cells are able to move to tumor sites where they can destroy cancer cells with cytotoxic enzyme (granzyme B) or cytokines (TNF-alpha or IFN-gamma). Since PD-L1 (B7-H1) expressed by tumors suppresses this process (Dong and Chen 2003), PD-L1 blockade is required to improve this antitumor immunity. Successful immunity will lead to another round of immune response by releasing more tumor antigens through destruction of tumor cells. This process is called the cancer-immunity cycle (Chen and Mellman 2013), describing the sequence of events in priming, expansion, and effector phases of T-cell responses to tumors.

Improving Antigen-Presentation to Prime More Immune Cells

Activation of the immune system to bring therapeutic benefit to cancer patients has been the subject of more than 100 years of study. Dr. Coley is believed to be the first physician to perform clinical trials in the treatment of cancer patients using dead bacteria (Coley 1906). His idea was that a strong immune response triggered by pathogens that can cure an infection would be able to cure a cancer as well. Thus, the so-called Coley's toxin was originally used as a trigger of the immune system to treat human cancer. Most of his trials failed, but occasionally some of his cancer patients experienced tumor regression. From his pioneering work on cancer immunotherapy, immunologists have learned the immuno-stimulatory power of his "toxin" and dissected its effective components to discover new functions of immune adjuvants (enhancers). These adjuvants have been tested to help immune responses to tumor vaccination. For example, the dead bacteria bacille Calmette-Guérin (BCG) that causes tuberculosis has been successfully used in the treatment of human bladder cancer. BCG is used to induce inflammatory cytokine production, therefore increasing efficiency of tumor antigen presentation from dead tumor cells.

Some defined tumor antigens or irradiated tumor cells can be used as vaccines in combination with certain powerful adjuvants to prevent tumor growth. Most human tumor antigens are normal, unmutated proteins that are aberrantly expressed on tumors. For example, gp100 and MART-1 tumor antigens are human melanoma tumor antigens, mainly expressed by melanoma cells rather than by normal cells. They are real tumor antigens because they can induce an immune response against the melanoma cells expressing them. However, these antigens need to be presented to immune cells by professional APCs. This requirement prompted the study of dendritic cell (DC) therapy using dendritic cells as APCs to present tumor antigen vaccines. The dendritic cells can be isolated from a patient's blood, loaded with the tumor antigen, and then re-injected into patients. Currently DC therapy is a complicated, costly procedure, but could be streamlined in combination with other immunotherapy. Besides tumor antigen-based vaccine therapy, viruses have been used as a new strategy to treat human cancers. Viruses that can attack tumor cells and cause them to die are called oncolytic viruses and have been selected for this treatment. Oncolytic viral therapy not only directly destroys the infected tumor cells, but also releases inflammatory mediators and tumor antigens that would further induce immune responses against the cancer.

Improving Immune Cell Expansion and Differentiation

Following activation by tumor antigens, T cells undergo proliferation either before or after they enter tumor sites. During this expansion period, they need additional signals to maintain their proliferation and to gain effector functions. To that purpose circulating proteins called cytokines provide them with the needed stimulation. Among them, interleukin 2 (IL-2) is an important factor for T cells to expand and become effector cells. The drug form of IL-2 (Proleukin®, aldesleukin) has been approved to treat human melanoma and kidney cancers based on their ability to help effector T cells to grow. However, the expansion of T cells is negatively controlled by the regulatory T cells (Treg). Before proliferation, T cells need to be activated. T-cell activation requires two signals—one is antigen stimulation through T-cell receptor (TCR), and the other is co-stimulation through CD28. CD28 receives signals from APCs by binding to B7 molecules expressed by APCs. Treg cells disrupt the interaction of CD28 and B7 by expressing CTLA-4 molecule because CTLA-4 has a higher affinity to binding B7 than CD28. Therefore, CTLA-4 can "out-compete" CD28 for binding and prevent co-stimulatory signals (Fig. 1.3). A current drug approved by the FDA in the treatment of cancer is ipilimumab (anti-CTLA-4). As an antibody to CTLA-4, it will block the function of CTLA-4 and prevent it from competing with CD28, resulting in more T-cell activation and expansion to fight cancers.

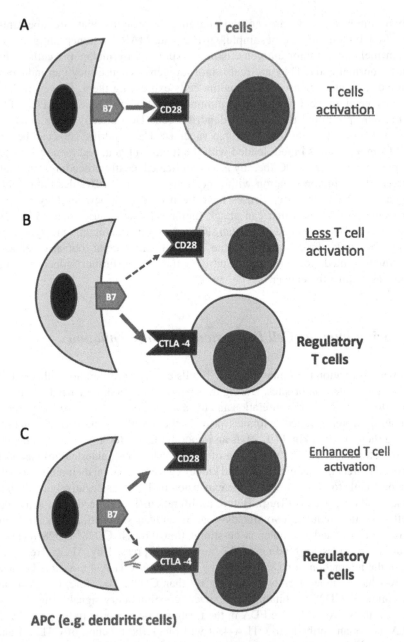

Fig. 1.3 (**a**) Antigen-presenting cells (APCs) use B7 to co-stimulate CD28 on T cells and activate them upon antigen stimulation. (**b**) Regulatory T cells have CTLA-4, which competes for B7 on the APCs, reducing the activation of T cells. (**c**) A blocking antibody to CTLA-4 can block CTLA-4 and let more B7 to interact with CD28, enhancing T-cell activation

Protecting Immune Cells from Suppressive Mechanisms Within Tumor Tissues

As mentioned above, once T cells are activated by antigen stimulation, they express high levels of PD-1, a receptor for transmitting signals that impede the function of T cells. While PD-1 expression could be good to prevent damage to healthy tissues or organs caused by over-activated T cells, PD-1 also restrains the antitumor activity of T cells. Tumor-reactive T cells tend to express high levels of PD-1 because they are continually exposed to tumor antigens in the tumor microenvironment. After such a long time of antigen stimulation, T cells become "exhausted." The hallmarks of exhausted T cells are weak function and poor survival. When PD-1 positive T cells come to tumor sites, their PD-1 will be engaged by PD-L1 expressed by most cancer cells. PD-L1 is a ligand of PD-1 and functions to induce T-cell death or reduce the T cell's ability to kill tumor cells. However, some exhausted T cells can be invigorated to restore their antitumor function and protected from cell death by blocking this PD-1/PD-L1 interaction (Gibbons Johnson and Dong 2017).

PD-L1 expression by tumor cells is an important mechanism of tumor immune evasion (a process tumor cells use to escape immune attacks). One effector molecule produced by T cells to suppress tumor growth is IFN (interferon) gamma that can directly inhibit the proliferation of tumor cells by impairing their DNA duplication. Interestingly, yet-to-be killed tumor cells take up a small amount of IFN-gamma as an inducer of their PD-L1 expression (Dong et al. 2002). This process is called adaptive resistance of the tumor to cancer immunity, as tumor cells become resistant to T-cell attacks when tumor cells increase their expression of PD-L1, which can disarm any T cells that approach (Taube et al. 2014). Not only do tumor cells express PD-L1, but some immune cells also express this ligand. APCs like dendritic cells and macrophages are known to express PD-L1. Since APCs play a key role in T-cell activation, they may use PD-L1 to restrain the degree of T-cell activation in order to prevent over-activation of T cells (Gibbons Johnson and Dong 2017). While it would be obvious that PD-L1 expression in human cancers may be useful in predicting response to PD-1/PD-L1 blockade therapy, patients with PD-L1 negative cancers have also responded to the same therapy. This suggests that PD-L1 expressed by host cells may be a therapeutic target similar to the PD-L1 expressed by tumor cells. PD-L2 (also called B7-DC) is another ligand of PD-1 (Tseng et al. 2001; Latchman et al. 2001). PD-L2 is not expressed by most human cancer cells, but is expressed by dendritic cells that infiltrate tumor tissues. Thus, PD-L2 expression could also be considered as a marker to evaluate the responsiveness to anti-PD-1 therapy. Besides PD-1 and PD-L1/2 pathways, many other immune checkpoint molecules (B7-H3, B7-H4, VISTA, PD-1H, Tim-3, LAG3, TIGIT, etc.) have been identified, and the therapeutic effects of blocking them have been tested in clinical trials (Yao et al. 2013). In the future, a rationalized and individualized combination of immune checkpoint blockade therapy could be formulated in one package that would fit individual cancer patients in order to improve the efficacy and reduce toxicity.

Adoptive T-Cell Transfer

As T cells are the final tumor killer cells, it has been speculated that injection of enough T cells into tumor sites would be able to reject tumors or suppress their growth. Since the early 1980s, T cells isolated from patients' tumors have been used to treat melanoma and kidney cancers (Rosenberg 2011). Recent technology allows us to expand T cells by thousands of times in culture dishes in a week or so. To increase the tumor-specificity of T cells, T cells are engineered to express receptors that are specific to tumor antigens present on the surface of tumor cells. These engineered T cells are called chimeric antigen receptor (CAR)-engineered T cells (CAR-T cells). Adoptive CAR-T cell transfer has achieved promising therapeutic effects in the control of some blood cancers. However, CAR-T cell therapy faces challenges in treatment of solid cancers as the transferred T cells may disappear rapidly if the tumor burden is large and may cause adverse effects in patients. More research is underway to improve its efficacy and safety.

Rational Combination in Cancer Therapy

Novel cancer immunotherapies targeting the immune checkpoint pathways have become a true paradigm shift in the treatment of patients with advanced cancers (Pardoll 2012), and are now the standard-of-care in seven different cancer types. However, only a small fraction of patients with solid cancers benefit from these immunotherapies with durable responses. One hurdle of cancer immunotherapy could be large tumor burdens. Strategies aimed to reduce tumor burden have the potential to promote efficacy or overcome resistance to cancer immunotherapy.

Radiation is known to trigger innate immune responses and impair immune suppressive cells. The potential of local radiation has been tested in many preclinical models to evaluate its ability to promote infiltration of tumor sites with effector T cells. To turn a local antitumor immune response to a systemic protection, additional methods are needed. Several clinical trials and preclinical studies have shown that administration of PD-1 or PD-L1 blockade can cause tumor regression in distant tumor sites that are not directly irradiated. This phenomenon is called the "abscopal effect" and suggests that immune cells primed at the irradiated sites would be able to circulate the whole body and find the same tumor cells and destroy them (Park et al. 2015). However, the optimal dose of irradiation and the timing of a combination of immune checkpoint inhibitors should be validated in future clinical trials.

The tumor cell death caused by certain chemotherapy agents provides a good source for releasing potential tumor-specific antigen proteins. This type of tumor cell death is called immunogenic cell death (ICD) (Obeid et al. 2007). In this regard, chemotherapy drugs that cause ICD could be used to "recharge" T cells by providing more tumor antigens that are released from dead tumor cells. This strategy could be very helpful in cancer patients who otherwise do not have spontaneous release of tumor antigens. Releasing these tumor antigens to activate T cells provides an opportunity for the addition of immune checkpoint blockade that can further improve the expansion of activated immune cells. This can help achieve a good number of activated immune cells to overcome the resistance caused by the overwhelming numbers of cancer cells. Based on this potential synergy effect, the FDA recently approved the combined therapy of chemotherapy and immunotherapy to treat lung cancers.

Prospects of Cancer Immunotherapy

Cancer immunotherapy is a personalized medicine because each patient has his or her own unique immune responses to cancer. The uniqueness of immune responses to cancer is not only determined by the diversity and specificity of our immune system in presentation and recognition of tumor antigens, but also by the heterogeneity of cancer antigens within each patient. The future of cancer immunotherapy should be a rational combined therapy that will meet the specific needs of each patient. While this task is not easy and could be very costly, it is the goal we should to strive for. To achieve this objective, scientifically we need to address several fundamental questions in tumor antigen presentation, T-cell function, and regulatory mechanisms, and clinically we need to address the optimal dose and sequences of immunotherapy drugs and to define mechanisms of drug resistance. We also need biomarkers to identify and evaluate the tumor-reactive T-cell responses in cancer patients in order to predict and monitor patient responses to immunotherapy.

Finally, after reading through all these technical terms and explanations, you may have a question for me: what can I do to improve my own immunity to cancer? Although cancer immunologists can give you a list of ways in which to do that, I would suggest getting enough sleep. While we are waiting for scientific validation of my answer, I hope you did not doze off when you were reading this chapter. But if this chapter really helps you sleep, I would love to know that.

References

Bunt, S. K., Sinha, P., Clements, V. K., Leips, J., & Ostrand-Rosenberg, S. (2006). Inflammation induces myeloid-derived suppressor cells that facilitate tumor progression. *Journal of Immunology, 176*(1), 284–290.

Casares, N., Arribillaga, L., Sarobe, P., Dotor, J., Lopez-Diaz de Cerio, A., Melero, I., Prieto, J., Borras-Cuesta, F., & Lasarte, J. J. (2003). CD4+/CD25+ regulatory cells inhibit activation of tumor-primed CD4+ T cells with IFN-gamma-dependent antiangiogenic activity, as well as long-lasting tumor immunity elicited by peptide vaccination. *Journal of Immunology, 171*(11), 5931–5939.

Chen, D. S., & Mellman, I. (2013). Oncology meets immunology: The cancer-immunity cycle. *Immunity, 39*(1), 1–10. https://doi.org/10.1016/j.immuni.2013.07.012.

Coley. (1906). Late results of the treatment of inoperable sarcoma by the mixed toxins of erysipelas and bacillus prodigiosus. *The American Journal of the Medical Sciences, 131*, 375–430.

Curiel, T. J., Coukos, G., Zou, L., Alvarez, X., Cheng, P., Mottram, P., Evdemon-Hogan, M., Conejo-Garcia, J. R., Zhang, L., Burow, M., Zhu, Y., Wei, S., Kryczek, I., Daniel, B., Gordon, A., Myers, L., Lackner, A., Disis, M. L., Knutson, K. L., Chen, L., & Zou, W. (2004). Specific recruitment of regulatory T cells in ovarian carcinoma fosters immune privilege and predicts reduced survival. *Nature Medicine, 10*(9), 942–949. https://doi.org/10.1038/nm1093.

Dong, H., & Chen, L. (2003). B7-H1 pathway and its role in the evasion of tumor immunity. *Journal of Molecular Medicine, 81*(5), 281–287. https://doi.org/10.1007/s00109-003-0430-2.

Dong, H., Strome, S. E., Salomao, D. R., Tamura, H., Hirano, F., Flies, D. B., Roche, P. C., Lu, J., Zhu, G., Tamada, K., Lennon, V. A., Celis, E., & Chen, L. (2002). Tumor-associated B7-H1 promotes T-cell apoptosis: A potential mechanism of immune evasion. *Nature Medicine, 8*(8), 793–800. https://doi.org/10.1038/nm730 nm730 [pii].

Dong, H., Zhu, G., Tamada, K., & Chen, L. (1999). B7-H1, a third member of the B7 family, co-stimulates T-cell proliferation and interleukin-10 secretion. *Nature Medicine, 5*(12), 1365–1369. https://doi.org/10.1038/70932.

Freeman, G. J., Long, A. J., Iwai, Y., Bourque, K., Chernova, T., Nishimura, H., Fitz, L. J., Malenkovich, N., Okazaki, T., Byrne, M. C., Horton, H. F., Fouser, L., Carter, L., Ling, V., Bowman, M. R., Carreno, B. M., Collins, M., Wood, C. R., & Honjo, T. (2000). Engagement of the PD-1 immunoinhibitory receptor by a novel B7 family member leads to negative regulation of lymphocyte activation. *The Journal of Experimental Medicine, 192*(7), 1027–1034.

Friberg, M., Jennings, R., Alsarraj, M., Dessureault, S., Cantor, A., Extermann, M., Mellor, A. L., Munn, D. H., & Antonia, S. J. (2002). Indoleamine 2,3-dioxygenase contributes to tumor cell evasion of T cell-mediated rejection. *International Journal of Cancer, 101*(2), 151–155. https://doi.org/10.1002/ijc.10645.

Gibbons Johnson, R. M., & Dong, H. (2017). Functional Expression of Programmed Death-Ligand 1 (B7-H1) by Immune Cells and Tumor Cells. *Frontiers in Immunology, 8*, 961. https://doi.org/10.3389/fimmu.2017.00961.

Greenman, C., Stephens, P., Smith, R., Dalgliesh, G. L., Hunter, C., Bignell, G., Davies, H., Teague, J., Butler, A., Stevens, C., Edkins, S., O'Meara, S., Vastrik, I., Schmidt, E. E., Avis, T., Barthorpe, S., Bhamra, G., Buck, G., Choudhury, B., Clements, J., Cole, J., Dicks, E., Forbes, S., Gray, K., Halliday, K., Harrison, R., Hills, K., Hinton, J., Jenkinson, A., Jones, D., Menzies, A., Mironenko, T., Perry, J., Raine, K., Richardson, D., Shepherd, R., Small, A., Tofts, C., Varian, J., Webb, T., West, S., Widaa, S., Yates, A., Cahill, D. P., Louis, D. N., Goldstraw, P., Nicholson, A. G., Brasseur, F., Looijenga, L., Weber, B. L., Chiew, Y. E., DeFazio, A., Greaves, M. F., Green, A. R., Campbell, P., Birney, E., Easton, D. F., Chenevix-Trench, G., Tan, M. H., Khoo, S. K., Teh, B. T., Yuen, S. T., Leung, S. Y., Wooster, R., Futreal, P. A., & Stratton, M. R. (2007). Patterns of somatic mutation in human cancer genomes. *Nature, 446*(7132), 153–158. https://doi.org/10.1038/nature05610.

Hellstrom, I., Hellstrom, K. E., Pierce, G. E., & Yang, J. P. (1968). Cellular and humoral immunity to different types of human neoplasms. *Nature, 220*(5174), 1352–1354.

Ishida, Y., Agata, Y., Shibahara, K., & Honjo, T. (1992). Induced expression of PD-1, a novel member of the immunoglobulin gene superfamily, upon programmed cell death. *The EMBO Journal, 11*(11), 3887–3895.

Iwai, Y., Ishida, M., Tanaka, Y., Okazaki, T., Honjo, T., & Minato, N. (2002). Involvement of PD-L1 on tumor cells in the escape from host immune system and tumor immunotherapy by PD-L1 blockade. *Proceedings of the National Academy of Sciences of the United States of America, 99*(19), 12293–12297. https://doi.org/10.1073/pnas.192461099.

Korman, A. J., Peggs, K. S., & Allison, J. P. (2006). Checkpoint blockade in cancer immunotherapy. *Advances in Immunology, 90*, 297–339. https://doi.org/10.1016/S0065-2776(06)90008-X.

Latchman, Y., Wood, C. R., Chernova, T., Chaudhary, D., Borde, M., Chernova, I., Iwai, Y., Long, A. J., Brown, J. A., Nunes, R., Greenfield, E. A., Bourque, K., Boussiotis, V. A., Carter, L. L., Carreno, B. M., Malenkovich, N., Nishimura, H., Okazaki, T., Honjo, T., Sharpe, A. H., &

Freeman, G. J. (2001). PD-L2 is a second ligand for PD-1 and inhibits T cell activation. *Nature Immunology, 2*(3), 261–268. https://doi.org/10.1038/85330.

Leach, D. R., Krummel, M. F., & Allison, J. P. (1996). Enhancement of antitumor immunity by CTLA-4 blockade. *Science, 271*(5256), 1734–1736.

Obeid, M., Tesniere, A., Ghiringhelli, F., Fimia, G. M., Apetoh, L., Perfettini, J. L., Castedo, M., Mignot, G., Panaretakis, T., Casares, N., Metivier, D., Larochette, N., van Endert, P., Ciccosanti, F., Piacentini, M., Zitvogel, L., & Kroemer, G. (2007). Calreticulin exposure dictates the immunogenicity of cancer cell death. *Nature Medicine, 13*(1), 54–61. https://doi.org/10.1038/nm1523.

Pardoll, D. M. (2012). The blockade of immune checkpoints in cancer immunotherapy. *Nature Reviews Cancer, 12*(4), 252–264. https://doi.org/10.1038/nrc3239.

Park, S. S., Dong, H., Liu, X., Harrington, S. M., Krco, C. J., Grams, M. P., Mansfield, A. S., Furutani, K. M., Olivier, K. R., & Kwon, E. D. (2015). PD-1 restrains radiotherapy-induced abscopal effect. *Cancer Immunology Research, 3*(6), 610–619. https://doi.org/10.1158/2326-6066.CIR-14-0138.

Rosenberg, S. A. (2011). Cell transfer immunotherapy for metastatic solid cancer – what clinicians need to know. *Nature Reviews. Clinical Oncology, 8*(10), 577–585. https://doi.org/10.1038/nrclinonc.2011.116.

Taube, J. M., Klein, A. P., Brahmer, J. R., Xu, H., Pan, X., Kim, J. H., Chen, L., Pardoll, D. M., Topalian, S. L., & Anders, R. A. (2014). Association of PD-1, PD-1 ligands, and other features of the tumor immune microenvironment with response to anti-PD-1 therapy. *Clinical Cancer Research*. https://doi.org/10.1158/1078-0432.CCR-13-3271

Thompson, R. H., Kuntz, S. M., Leibovich, B. C., Dong, H., Lohse, C. M., Webster, W. S., Sengupta, S., Frank, I., Parker, A. S., Zincke, H., Blute, M. L., Sebo, T. J., Cheville, J. C., & Kwon, E. D. (2006). Tumor B7-H1 is associated with poor prognosis in renal cell carcinoma patients with long-term follow-up. *Cancer Research, 66*(7), 3381–3385. doi:66/7/3381 [pii]. https://doi.org/10.1158/0008-5472.CAN-05-4303

Tomasetti, C., Li, L., & Vogelstein, B. (2017). Stem cell divisions, somatic mutations, cancer etiology, and cancer prevention. *Science, 355*(6331), 1330–1334. https://doi.org/10.1126/science.aaf9011.

Tseng, D., Volkmer, J. P., Willingham, S. B., Contreras-Trujillo, H., Fathman, J. W., Fernhoff, N. B., Seita, J., Inlay, M. A., Weiskopf, K., Miyanishi, M., & Weissman, I. L. (2013). Anti-CD47 antibody-mediated phagocytosis of cancer by macrophages primes an effective antitumor T-cell response. *Proceedings of the National Academy of Sciences of the United States of America, 110*(27), 11103–11108. https://doi.org/10.1073/pnas.1305569110.

Tseng, S. Y., Otsuji, M., Gorski, K., Huang, X., Slansky, J. E., Pai, S. I., Shalabi, A., Shin, T., Pardoll, D. M., & Tsuchiya, H. (2001). B7-DC, a new dendritic cell molecule with potent costimulatory properties for T cells. *The Journal of Experimental Medicine, 193*(7), 839–846.

van der Bruggen, P., Traversari, C., Chomez, P., Lurquin, C., De Plaen, E., Van den Eynde, B., Knuth, A., & Boon, T. (1991). A gene encoding an antigen recognized by cytolytic T lymphocytes on a human melanoma. *Science, 254*(5038), 1643–1647.

Yao, S., Zhu, Y., & Chen, L. (2013). Advances in targeting cell surface signalling molecules for immune modulation. *Nature Reviews. Drug Discovery, 12*(2), 130–146. https://doi.org/10.1038/nrd3877.

Chapter 2
Therapeutic Targets of FDA-Approved Immunotherapies in Oncology

Svetomir N. Markovic and Anagha Bangalore Kumar

Contents

Introduction

Cancer is a leading cause of death in the industrialized world second only to cardiovascular diseases. It is estimated that the number of people living with cancer is increasing. The most commonly diagnosed malignancy in women is breast cancer and that in men is prostate cancer. Lung cancer and colorectal cancer are the second and third most commonly diagnosed cancers, respectively, in both men and women (Siegel et al. 2015). Cancer immunotherapy aims to augment the patient's own immune system, especially T cells, to fight cancer. In recent years cancer immunotherapy (otherwise referred as immuno-oncology, IO) has emerged to be a promising modality in cancer treatment (Mellman et al. 2011). Numerous agents have received US Food and Drug Administration (FDA) approval to treat patients, with

S.N. Markovic (✉)
Department of Oncology, Department of Medicine/Division of Hematology,
Department of Immunology, College of Medicine, Mayo Clinic, Rochester, MN, USA

A.B. Kumar
Clinical Pharmacology Fellow, Mayo Clinic, Rochester, MN, USA

© Springer International Publishing AG 2018
H. Dong, S.N. Markovic (eds.), *The Basics of Cancer Immunotherapy*,
https://doi.org/10.1007/978-3-319-70622-1_2

seemingly ever-increasing efficacy. Herein we summarize the state of the art of FDA-approved agents used in clinical practice that aim to achieve a therapeutic benefit by modulating pre-existing anti-tumor immunity (Table 2.1).

Table 2.1 Summary of the US Food and Drug Administration (FDA)-approved monoclonal antibodies used in oncology

Drug	Target	Immunological relevance	FDA-approved indication	Side effects
Alemtuzumab	CD 52, humanized	CD 52 is expressed on mature lymphocytes, monocytes, and dendritic cells	Chronic lymphocytic lymphoma, cutaneous T-cell lymphoma	Rash, headache, hyper-/ hypothyroidism, infections, infusion reaction (Black box warning—cytopenia and infusion reaction, infection)
Ado-trastuzumab	HER2, humanized, conjugated with drug emtansine	HER2 is a member of human epidermal growth factor receptor family facilitates uncontrolled cell growth and angiogenesis	HER2-positive breast cancer	Tiredness, nausea, bleeding, infusion reactions (Black box warning—cardiac toxicity, hepatotoxicity, fetal death or birth defects)
Atezolizumab	PD-L-inhibitor, humanized	PD-L1 binding to PD-1 releases inhibitory stimuli for T-cell activation, proliferation, and survival	Non-squamous cell lung cancer (NSCLC)	Immune-related effects, nausea, fatigue, infections
Avelumab	PD-L1 inhibitor, human	PD-L1 binding to PD-1 releases inhibitory stimuli for T-cell activation, proliferation, and survival	Merkel cell carcinoma	Immune-related side effects, nausea, rash
Bevacizumab	VEGF-A, recombinant, humanized	VEGF-A receptor plays a role in angiogenesis, endothelial cell growth, encourages cell migration and inhibits apoptosis	Colorectal cancer, non-squamous, non-small-cell lung cancer, breast cancer, metastatic renal cell carcinoma, glioblastoma multiforme, ovarian, fallopian tube or peritoneal cancer, cervical cancer	Hypertension, bleeding, infection, worsens coronary artery disease and peripheral arterial disease (Black box warning—gastrointestinal perforation, wound dehiscence, wound-healing problems)

(continued)

Table 2.1 (continued)

Drug	Target	Immunological relevance	FDA-approved indication	Side effects
Blinatumomab	CD 19, murine	CD 19 is expressed on follicular dendritic cells and B cells. B cells lose it on maturation to plasma cells	Relapsed or refractory B-cell precursor, acute lymphoblastic leukemia	Agitation, swelling of extremities and face, blurred vision, chest pain, fever (Black box warning—neurological toxicities, cytokine release syndrome)
Brentuximab	CD 30 chimeric, conjugated with drug Auristatin E	Tumor marker on Reed Sternberger cell and anaplastic lymphoma	Hodgkin's lymphoma, anaplastic large cell lymphoma	Peripheral neuropathy, neutropenia, fatigue, nausea (Black box warning—probably fatal, progressive multifocal leukoencephalopathy (PML) due to viral infections)
Daratumumab	CD 38, human	CD 38 is expressed on immune cells like CD4, CD 8, B cells, and natural killer cells. It plays a role in cell adhesion, signal transduction, and calcium signaling	Multiple myeloma	Infusion reaction, fatigue, nausea, anemia, thrombocytopenia
Durvalumab	PD-L1 inhibitor, human	PD-L1 binding to PD-1 releases inhibitory stimuli for T-cell activation, proliferation, and survival	Urothelial cancer	Fatigue, musculoskeletal pain, constipation, swelling of extremities
Elotuzumab	CD 319, humanized	CD 319 is expressed on normal and malignant plasma cells	Multiple myeloma	Fatigue, diarrhea, nausea, fever
Ibritumomab	CD 20 murine, conjugated with Yttrium[90] or Indium[111]	CD 20 is expressed on B cells from pro-B-cell phase to memory cells but not plasma cells	Non-Hodgkin's lymphoma	Hypertension, low blood counts, rash, infusion reaction, infections (Black box warning—cytopenia and infusion reaction)

(continued)

Table 2.1 (continued)

Drug	Target	Immunological relevance	FDA-approved indication	Side effects
Ipilimumab	CTLA-4, human	CTLA-4 protein is present on T cell, functions as an immune checkpoint. When bound to CD 80/CD 86 on antigen presenting cells, it acts as an off-switch and downregulates T-cell activation and proliferation	Melanoma	Immunological side effects, diarrhea, demyelination
Nivolumab	PD-1 checkpoint inhibitor	PD-1 acts as an immune checkpoint. PD-L1 binding to PD-1 releases inhibitory stimuli for T-cell activation, proliferation, and survival	Advanced melanoma, lung cancer, head and neck squamous cell cancers, lung cancer, Hodgkin's lymphoma, renal cell carcinoma	Immune-mediated inflammation of lungs, colon, liver, kidney, rash
Obinutuzumab	CD 20 humanized	CD 20 is expressed on B cells from pro-B-cell phase to memory cells but not plasma cells	Chronic lymphocytic leukemia	Progressive multifocal leukoencephalopathy (PML), reactivation of hepatitis B, infusion reaction, bleeding (Black box warning—hepatitis B reactivation, PML)
Ofatumumab	CD 20, human	CD 20 is expressed on B cells from pro-B-cell phase to memory cells but not plasma cells	Chronic lymphocytic leukemia	Rash, pancytopenia, infections
Pembrolizumab	PD-1	PD-1 acts as an immune checkpoint. PD-L1 binding to PD-1 releases inhibitory stimuli for T-cell activation, proliferation, and survival	Metastatic melanoma, NSCLC, head and neck SCC	Immune-related inflammation of endocrine organs, lungs, kidney, rash, fatigue, infections

(continued)

Table 2.1 (continued)

Drug	Target	Immunological relevance	FDA-approved indication	Side effects
Pertuzumab	HER2, humanized	HER2 is a member of human epidermal growth factor receptor family, facilitates uncontrolled cell growth and angiogenesis	HER2-positive, locally advanced, inflammatory, early-stage breast cancer	Diarrhea, infection, rash, headache (Black box warning—fetal death, birth defects)
Ramucirumab	VEGFR2, human	VEGF receptor plays a role in angiogenesis, endothelial cell growth, encourages cell migration, and inhibits apoptosis	Advanced gastric or gastroesophageal junction adenocarcinoma, metastatic NSCLC, metastatic CRC	Diarrhea, hyponatremia, headache, high BP (Black box warning—gastrointestinal perforation, wound dehiscence, wound-healing problems)
Rituximab	CD 20, chimeric	CD 20 is expressed on B cells from pro-B-cell phase to memory cells but not plasma cells	Diffuse large B-cell lymphoma, non-Hodgkin's lymphoma, chronic lymphocytic lymphoma	Infusion reaction, cardiac arrest, cytokine arrest syndrome, tumor lysis syndrome, infections (Black box warning—infusion reaction, probably fatal PML due to viral infections and infections)
Siltuximab	IL-6, chimeric	IL-6 is a cytokine with both proinflammatory and anti-inflammatory properties	HIV and HHV8-negative Castleman's disease	Edema, arthralgia, infections
Trastuzumab	HER2, humanized	HER2 is a member of human epidermal growth factor receptor family, facilitates uncontrolled cell growth and angiogenesis	HER2-positive gastric or gastrointestinal tumors, breast cancer	Flu-like symptoms, nausea, diarrhea, cardiac toxicity (Black box warning— infusion reaction and cytopenia, cardiotoxicity)

Immune System and Cancer

The interplay between the immune system and cancer is complex. At the inception of a malignancy, according to our current understanding of cancer immunity, the immune system attempts to destroy cancer cells that are identified as a foreign. This is the first or "elimination phase." However, due to the heterogeneity among cancer cells, some of them escape this phase and enter the "equilibrium phase," in which they undergo mutations that further help them survive, while undetected by the host immune response. This phase is characterized by a continuous process of mutations and modifications to enable tumor cells to survive escaping the host immunity. This process is also called "cancer immunoediting." By the time these tumor cells enter the "escape phase," they have become resistant to immune control, and grow progressively as tumor masses (Smyth et al. 2006; Dunn et al. 2004). Furthermore, tumors escape immune recognition by presenting as a self-antigen, undergoing antigenic modulation, creating a state of immune suppression, creating a physical barrier from immune cells, or expressing antigens with low immunogenicity (Beatty and Gladney 2015).

An anti-cancer immune response requires a series of events to occur effectively:

(a) The tumor antigens are picked up by the antigen-presenting dendritic cells.
(b) Dendritic cells present the antigen to T cells on MHC class I and/or class II molecules.
(c) Effective "presentation" of tumor antigens from dendritic cells to effector/regulatory T cells capable of destroying cancer cells.
(d) Trafficking of effector cytotoxic (killer) T cells that reach the tumors and bind to the specific tumor antigen-expressing cancer cells and destroy them.

This cycle of events is actively disturbed in patients with cancer through many different mechanisms, including: (i) the immune system might fail to detect the tumor antigen, (ii) dendritic cells and T cells might treat the tumor antigen as a self-antigen, (iii) effector T cells might not be able to infiltrate the tumor, or (iv) the tumor microenvironment might inhibit the production of effector T cells (Motz and Coukos 2013; Chen and Mellman 2013). Cancer immunotherapy aims to redirect this natural cycle of tumor immunity. Careful regulation of this therapy is essential to avoid severe adverse effects.

Overview of Available Immunotherapies

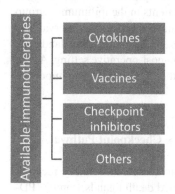

Immune Checkpoint Inhibitors

Cytotoxic T-Lymphocyte Associated Protein 4 (CTLA-4)

CTLA-4 is a member of the CD 28:B7 immunoglobulin family and is normally expressed in low levels on naïve effector T cells and regulatory T cells. After stimulation, CTLA-4 competes with CD 28 to bind with B7. When CTLA-4 binds with B7, it turns off the T-cell receptor signaling (Linsley et al. 1996). It plays an important role in preventing autoimmunity by downregulating T-cell activation (Peggs et al. 2006). Ipilimumab is an anti-CTLA-4 antibody that causes blockade of CTLA-4 resulting in prolonged T-cell activation, proliferation, and anti-tumor response (Peggs et al. 2006).

Ipilimumab, an antibody that targets CTLA-4, was the first checkpoint inhibitor approved for cancer treatment. It is being used successfully in the clinic. Hodi et al. compared ipilimumab and gp100 vaccine (control) in their phase 3 study consisting of 676 patients with melanoma. They randomized the group in a 3:1:1 ratio consisting of 403 patients receiving ipilimumab plus gp100, 137 patients receiving only ipilimumab, and 136 patients receiving only gp100. Patients received 3 mg/kg for 3 weeks up to four doses with or without gp100. The median overall survival was 10.0 months among patients receiving ipilimumab plus gp100, as compared with 6.4 months among patients receiving gp100 alone. There was no difference in overall survival (Hodi et al. 2010) This study led to FDA approval of the drug for metastatic melanoma. Robert et al. conducted another phase 3 trial on melanoma patients using ipilimumab 10 mg/kg plus dacarbazine comparing it with placebo plus dacarbazine. Ipilimumab or the placebo was administered at weeks 1, 4, 7, and 10 with dacarbazine, followed by dacarbazine alone once in 3 weeks till 22 weeks. The median overall survival in the ipilimumab group was 11.2 months versus 9.1 months in the placebo group (Robert et al. 2011) Patients with surgically resected, high risk of relapse melanoma were treated postoperatively with ipilimumab (10 mg/kg) or placebo. This was a phase 3 clinical trial with 476 patients in the ipilimumab group versus 476 patients in the placebo group. The median recurrence-free interval was significantly higher in the ipilimumab group (26.1 vs. 17.1 months). This landmark study led to the approval of the drug in adjuvant or the post-operative setting. As the first checkpoint inhibitor approved in melanoma by the FDA, it marks an important milestone in cancer therapy.

Programmed Cell Death Protein 1 (PD-1) Immune Checkpoint Pathway

Programmed cell death protein 1 (PD-1) belongs to the co-stimulatory receptor family of B7-CD28. It binds to its ligands programmed death ligands 1 and 2 (PD-L1 and PD-L2) and downregulates T-cell activation. PD-1 binding inhibits T-cell activation and reduces cytokine production and T-cell survival (Chen and Mellman 2013; Dong et al. 1999; Sharpe et al. 2007). Drugs targeting this pathway help in reactivating T cells to provide anti-tumoral responses.

Pembrolizumab is a PD-1 inhibitor that has been approved for use in melanoma, non-squamous cell lung cancer (NSCLC), and head and neck cancers. It is showing promising results in the clinic. It was administered in advanced melanoma patients at a dose of 10 mg/kg every 2 or 3 weeks or 2 mg/kg every 3 weeks. A total of 137 patients were treated and the response was assessed. The median progression-free interval was 7 months in advanced melanoma (Hamid et al. 2013). Pembrolizumab was the first PD-1 checkpoint inhibitor approved by the FDA for unresectable or metastatic melanoma. In another phase 3 trial, Robert et al. compared pembrolizumab and ipilimumab. They included 834 melanoma patients randomized in a ratio of 1:1:1 to receive pembrolizumab 10 mg/kg every 2 weeks, every 3 weeks, and ipilimumab 3 mg/kg every 3 weeks for four cycles. They reported the progression-free interval was much higher with pembrolizumab than with ipilimumab. The difference in dose of pembrolizumab did not change the efficacy of the drug. The adverse effects were also fewer in the pembrolizumab group (Robert et al. 2015). Pembrolizumab was also approved for NSCLC. Reck et al. compared pembrolizumab with chemotherapy in 301 patients with NSCLC expressing PD-1. They reported longer progression-free interval and overall survival and fewer side effects in the pembrolizumab group compared to chemotherapy (Reck et al. 2016). Pembrolizumab achieved accelerated approval for head and neck cancer after a study found a high response rate. At present, phase 3 trials are ongoing.

Nivolumab is a PD-1 inhibitor approved for melanoma, renal cell carcinoma (RCC), NSCLC, and head and neck squamous cell carcinoma after success in the clinic (Larkin et al. 2017; Tomita et al. 2017; Long et al. 2017; Brahmer et al. 2015, Harrington et al. 2017). Similarly, Durvalumab is approved for urothelial cancer, avelumab for Merkel cell carcinoma, and atezolizumab for NSCLC.

Checkpoint inhibitors are associated with an interesting spectrum of immune-mediated side effects. Immune-mediated side effects can target the skin, endocrine system, liver, gastrointestinal tract, nervous system, eyes, respiratory system, and hematopoietic system. CTLA4 inhibitors are frequently associated with colitis/diarrhea, dermatitis, hepatitis, and endocrinopathies. Fatigue, rash, and diarrhea are common side effects of PD1 inhibitors.

Therapy Targeting the Tumor Microenvironment

The immune cells in the tumor microenvironment play a role in protecting the tumors. It is predicted that the interaction between the tumor cells and their microenvironment protects them from traditional anti-cancer drugs. In multiple myeloma, junctions are formed between the myeloma cells and bone marrow stromal cells. These junctions play a role in signaling between the myeloma and stromal cells thus protecting them (Hideshima et al. 2004). Elotuzumab is a monoclonal antibody against the signaling lymphocytic activation molecule F7 (SLAMF7) receptor. This antibody blocks the protective signals between myeloma cells and stromal cells (Magen and Muchtar 2016; Lonial et al. 2016). The FDA has approved its use with lenalidomide and dexamethasone. The results of monoclonal antibodies in cancer therapy are inspiring scientists to develop more anti-cancer antibodies.

Vaccines

Vaccines against human papilloma virus (HPV) and hepatitis B have been used successfully to prevent cancers caused by these infections. Harald zur Hausen was awarded the Nobel Prize in physiology and medicine for the discovery of the HPV vaccine to prevent cervical cancer (Nour 2009). Understanding the immune system and its role in cancer treatment encouraged early attempts to develop anti-cancer vaccines. However, early attempts to develop a vaccine that can prevent cancer did not produce fruitful results (Topalian et al. 2011; Mellman et al. 2011). Vaccines stimulate host immunity to fight cancer. They are easy to administer in the outpatient clinic and minimally toxic. However, lack of an ideal antigen to design a vaccine and poor efficacy are major drawbacks (Yaddanapudi et al. 2013).

An ideal anti-cancer vaccine must break the tolerance developed by tumor cells. Antigens can be targeted to be picked up by dendritic cells. Activated dendritic cells play an important role in coordinating between innate and adoptive responses and are capable of breaking tumor tolerance (Topalian et al. 2011; Palucka and Banchereau 2012). Various antigens were tried to activate the dendritic cells. An ideal antigen needed to activate dendritic cells would be expressed only on the tumor and not in normal tissue. They did not promise reliable results clinically (Rosenberg et al. 2004). Combination with other immunostimulants like IL-2 has given better results (Schwartzentruber et al. 2011). Melanoma antigen family 3 (MAGE-3) is a tumor-specific protein expressed in melanoma, NSCLC, hematological malignancies, etc. The vaccine is a fusion protein of MAGE-3 and Haemophilus influenza protein D. This MAGE-3-containing vaccine was tried in NSCLC, but without satisfactory clinical reports (Vansteenkiste et al. 2007). GVAX consists of whole tumor cells genetically modified to secrete cytokines and irradiated to prevent cell division. GVAX failed in phase 3 trials too, probably because the antigens could not activate the dendritic cells effectively (Copier and Dalgleish 2010).

Unsatisfactory results of cell-based vaccines led researchers to develop dendritic cell (DC)-based vaccines. Here, DCs are isolated from the patient's blood, activated with tumor antigen, and reinjected into the patient (Schuler 2010; Sabado and Bhardwaj 2013). These vaccines have given better clinical results. Sipuleucel-T is a DC-based vaccine that is developed with prostate acid phosphatase and DC growth factor and used for prostate cancer (Higano et al. 2009; Kantoff et al. 2010). It was approved by the FDA in 2010 (Farkona et al. 2016). A phase 3 trial successfully demonstrated prolonged overall survival in patients with metastatic castration resistant prostatic cancer who had received the vaccine compared to the control group. It increased the median survival by 4 months; however, there was no impressive reduction in tumor volume (Kantoff et al. 2010). One of the major advantages is that there is no risk of HLA mismatch. It is also relatively hard to prepare and administer (Mellman et al. 2011).

Intravesical bacillus Calmette-Guérin (BCG) is the only FDA-approved treatment for in situ bladder cancer.

Oncolytic Virus Therapy

Viruses can replicate in cancer cells and the viral genome can be modified to alter its virulence and increase anti-tumor activity. Promoters can be added into viral genes to reduce or delete the genes expressing pathogenicity (DeWeese et al. 2001; Brown et al. 1997). Also, some oncolytic virures can be designed to produce cytokines that are required for T-cell activation (Hu et al. 2006; Liu et al. 2003; Fukuhara et al. 2005). Tumor antigens are released after the virus kills the infected cells. Then, there is a specific CD 8 T-cell-mediated anti-tumor response that is mounted against these antigens (Kaufman et al. 2015). The challenge encountered in viral vaccines is the risk of the immune system recognizing the virus and clearing it from the body before it serves its purpose. This can be overcome by methods that prevent the virus being recognized as an antigen. Pegylation of the viral coat or genetically modifying the viral genome to inhibit antigen presentation are such methods (Tesfay et al. 2013).

Herpes simplex virus, measles virus, vaccinia virus, reovirus, Newcastle disease virus, and Seneca Valley virus have been tried for viral vaccines (Chiocca and Rabkin 2014). So far, the most promising one has been Talimogene laherparepvec

(T-VEC), a modified oncolytic herpes simplex virus type 1. The coding sequence for granulocyte macrophage colony-stimulating factor (GM-CSF) has been included in its genome and the ones for neuronal development have been deleted (Liu et al. 2003; Toda et al. 2000). This increases oncolytic therapeutic efficacy (Liu et al. 2003). A phase 3 trial was conducted enrolling 439 patients with unresectable melanoma. Patients were randomized in a 2:1 ratio to intralesional T-VEC or subcutaneous GM-CSF. T-VEC was injected into one or more tumor sites at a concentration of 10^8 plaque-forming units/ml on day 1 and day 15 of each 28-day cycle for 12 months. GM-CSF was administered at a dose of 125 $\mu g/m^2/day$ subcutaneously for the first 14 days of the 28-day cycle for 12 months. The study found that there was a better overall response rate in patients receiving T-VEC compared to those receiving GM-CSF (16.3 vs. 2.1, p-value < 0.001). The overall survival was also increased in those receiving T-VEC. The most common side effects were fever, fatigue, nausea, and reaction at the injection site. In October 2015, the FDA approved T-VEC to treat advanced melanoma (Kaufman and Bines 2010).

There are currently many clinical trials testing various anti-cancer vaccines. They are also being tried in combination with other approved drugs. There are several obstacles that have to be cleared before they get formal approval. Side-effect profile, cost, and efficacy are the main limitations of oncolytic virus therapy. Nevertheless, anti-cancer vaccines have potential scope in this field.

Cytokines

Cytokines are cell-signaling molecules that function as paracrine mediators of cell-cell interactions, secreted by one cell to influence the behaviors of another, usually closely approximated, cell. Cytokines exhibiting immune cell activation properties have been tested in oncology as potential immune-activating, anti-tumor drugs. It was hoped they would stimulate the host immune system providing durable anti-tumor responses. However, despite many tested agents, only a few have reached FDA approval for clinical use in oncology: interferons and interleukin- 2 (Lee and Margolin 2011).

Interferon-alfa (IFNα) inhibits the growth of virus-induced tumors and epithelial tumors. Interferons (IFNs) have antiproliferative, immunoregulatory, and antiviral properties (Li et al. 2009). IFNs have been tried in various malignancies with variable success rates (Platanias 2013; Stein and Tiu 2013). Jorge Quesada et al. utilized IFNα-A in advanced hairy cell leukemia. They used 3 million units daily and achieved remission of the disease (Quesada et al. 1986). It was then used to treat 30 patients with hairy cell leukemia and it was successful in achieving partial remission in 17 patients and complete remission in nine patients (Bonnem 1991; Vedantham et al. 1992). It was later approved by the FDA for this condition (Veronese and Mero 2008). In melanoma, it is a useful adjuvant therapy. Multiple studies have demonstrated an increase in relapse-free survival, with few suggesting a positive impact on overall survival, especially in a subset of patients presenting with ulcerated primary melanomas (Ascierto et al. 2014; Kirkwood et al. 2001; Mocellin et al. 2010; Pasquali and Mocellin 2010). Conjugation with polyethylene glycol seems to reduce the side effects without altering the efficacy. Pegylated IFNα was FDA-approved for metastatic melanoma in 2011 (Eggermont et al. 2008). It is associated with flu-like syndromes, nausea, dizziness, anorexia, and leukopenia (Daud et al. 2012). Its side effects limit its clinical use.

Interleukin-2 (IL-2) has pleiotropic effects on the immune system, and especially plays a role in T-cell and natural killer-cell activation (Morgan et al. 1976). It has been approved by the FDA for metastatic melanoma and RCC (Jiang et al. 2016). In an initial study with high-dose (HD) IL-2, four of seven patients with melanoma and all three cases of RCC showed response (Rosenberg et al. 1985). A phase 2 trial conducted on 255 patients with metastatic RCC using HD IL-2 had a response rate of 15% (Rosenberg 2014.) Although monotherapy with IL-2 was approved for RCC and melanoma, it did not improve overall survival in those patients. Combination with other anti-cancer treatments has been shown to improve its efficacy and reduce side effects. In a phase 3 trial in patients with RCC, HD IL-2 monotherapy had higher response rates than in those receiving low-dose IL-2 and IFNα (McDermott et al. 2005). Similarly, combination therapy with other chemotherapeutic agents has not given impressive results (Ives et al. 2007; Sasse et al. 2007). Combination with targeted inhibitors has increased the efficacy of these drugs (Chen et al. 1997; Bersanelli et al. 2014). A recent phase 3 trial compared HD IL-2 alone and IL-2 with gp 100 peptide vaccines (Schwartzentruber et al. 2011). It was reported that addition of IL-2 enhanced the efficacy of the vaccine in melanoma patients (Overwijk et al. 2000; Smith et al. 2008). HD IL-2 can be used as an adjuvant in melanoma therapy. IL-2 is associated with vascular leak syndrome, pulmonary edema, hypotension, and cardiotoxicity (Peace and Cheever 1989).

Combination Therapy

A number of cancer patients require more than a single agent to respond. Complete remission may require multiple drugs acting on different targets. Many immunotherapeutic agents have been tried in combination in cancer patients and some have yielded impressive results (Mahoney et al. 2015). CTLA-4 and PD1 inhibitors use different signaling pathways to activate T cells and have been used in combination (Topalian et al. 2011). The combined use of nivolumab and ipilimumab was approved for melanoma in 2015. As this combination enhances anti-tumor immunity, it also increases the adverse effects. Similarly, bevacizumab and IFNα have acquired FDA approval for combined use in RCC. Considering the vast array of immune-modifying agents available on the market and the even greater number of developing agents, the future of cancer immunotherapy will depend on the optimization of combination immunotherapeutics aiming to maximize anti-tumor efficacy and minimize treatment-related toxicity.

Conclusion

In the nineteenth century, William Coley first identified that the body's response to infections could have anti-tumor effects. He used a toxin made of bacteria to treat patients with cancer. This discovery and practice paved the way for modern immunotherapy. After decades of effort and dedication, scientists have developed various techniques to harness the immune system to fight cancer. There are multiple trials that have been currently launched to evaluate the products in the clinical setting. The discovery of checkpoint inhibitors has revolutionized modern oncology. There is still scope to develop combination therapies, biomarkers to predict response, and novel agents to achieve increased therapeutic success.

References

Ascierto, P. A., Chiarion-Sileni, V., Muggiano, A., Mandala, M., Pimpinelli, N., Del Vecchio, M., Rinaldi, G., Simeone, E., & Queirolo, P. (2014). Interferon alpha for the adjuvant treatment of melanoma: Review of international literature and practical recommendations from an expert panel on the use of interferon. *Journal of Chemotherapy, 26*, 193–201.

Beatty, G. L., & Gladney, W. L. (2015). Immune escape mechanisms as a guide for cancer immunotherapy. *Clinical Cancer Research, 21*, 687–692.

Bersanelli, M., Buti, S., Camisa, R., Brighenti, M., Lazzarelli, S., Mazza, G., & Passalacqua, R. (2014). Gefitinib plus interleukin-2 in advanced non-small cell lung cancer patients previously treated with chemotherapy. *Cancers (Basel), 6*, 2035–2048.

Bonnem, E. M. (1991). alpha Interferon: The potential drug of adjuvant therapy: Past achievements and future challenges. *European Journal of Cancer, 27*(Suppl 4), S2–S6.

Brahmer, J., Reckamp, K. L., Baas, P., Crino, L., Eberhardt, W. E., Poddubskaya, E., Antonia, S., Pluzanski, A., Vokes, E. E., Holgado, E., Waterhouse, D., Ready, N., Gainor, J., Aren Frontera, O., Havel, L., Steins, M., Garassino, M. C., Aerts, J. G., Domine, M., Paz-Ares, L., Reck, M., Baudelet, C., Harbison, C. T., Lestini, B., & Spigel, D. R. (2015). Nivolumab versus docetaxel in advanced squamous-cell non-small-cell lung cancer. *The New England Journal of Medicine, 373*, 123–135.

Brown, S. M., Maclean, A. R., Mckie, E. A., & Harland, J. (1997). The herpes simplex virus virulence factor ICP34.5 and the cellular protein MyD116 complex with proliferating cell nuclear antigen through the 63-amino-acid domain conserved in ICP34.5, MyD116, and GADD34. *Journal of Virology, 71*, 9442–9449.

Chen, D. S., & Mellman, I. (2013). Oncology meets immunology: The cancer-immunity cycle. *Immunity, 39*, 1–10.

Chen, Y. M., Yang, W. K., Whang-Peng, J., Tsai, W. Y., Hung, Y. M., Yang, D. M., Lin, W. C., Perng, R. P., & Ting, C. C. (1997). Restoration of the immunocompetence by IL-2 activation and TCR-CD3 engagement of the in vivo anergized tumor-specific CTL from lung cancer patients. *Journal of Immunotherapy, 20*, 354–364.

Chiocca, E. A., & Rabkin, S. D. (2014). Oncolytic viruses and their application to cancer immunotherapy. *Cancer Immunology Research, 2*, 295–300.

Copier, J., & Dalgleish, A. (2010). Whole-cell vaccines: A failure or a success waiting to happen? *Current Opinion in Molecular Therapeutics, 12*, 14–20.

Daud, A., Soon, C., Dummer, R., Eggermont, A. M., Hwu, W. J., Grob, J. J., Garbe, C., & Hauschild, A. (2012). Management of pegylated interferon alpha toxicity in adjuvant therapy of melanoma. *Expert Opinion on Biological Therapy, 12*, 1087–1099.

Deweese, T. L., Van Der Poel, H., Li, S., Mikhak, B., Drew, R., Goemann, M., Hamper, U., Dejong, R., Detorie, N., Rodriguez, R., Haulk, T., Demarzo, A. M., Piantadosi, S., Yu, D. C., Chen, Y., Henderson, D. R., Carducci, M. A., Nelson, W. G., & Simons, J. W. (2001). A phase I trial of CV706, a replication-competent, PSA selective oncolytic adenovirus, for the treatment of locally recurrent prostate cancer following radiation therapy. *Cancer Research, 61*, 7464–7472.

Dong, H., Zhu, G., Tamada, K., & Chen, L. (1999). B7-H1, a third member of the B7 family, co-stimulates T-cell proliferation and interleukin-10 secretion. *Nature Medicine, 5*, 1365–1369.

Dunn, G. P., Old, L. J., & Schreiber, R. D. (2004). The three Es of cancer immunoediting. *Annual Review of Immunology, 22*, 329–360.

Eggermont, A. M., Suciu, S., Santinami, M., Testori, A., Kruit, W. H., Marsden, J., Punt, C. J., Sales, F., Gore, M., Mackie, R., Kusic, Z., Dummer, R., Hauschild, A., Musat, E., Spatz, A., Keilholz, U., & GROUP, E. M. (2008). Adjuvant therapy with pegylated interferon alfa-2b versus observation alone in resected stage III melanoma: Final results of EORTC 18991, a randomised phase III trial. *Lancet, 372*, 117–126.

Farkona, S., Diamandis, E. P., & Blasutig, I. M. (2016). Cancer immunotherapy: The beginning of the end of cancer? *BMC Medicine, 14*, 73.

Fukuhara, H., Ino, Y., Kuroda, T., Martuza, R. L., & Todo, T. (2005). Triple gene-deleted oncolytic herpes simplex virus vector double-armed with interleukin 18 and soluble B7-1 constructed by bacterial artificial chromosome-mediated system. *Cancer Research, 65*, 10663–10668.

Hamid, O., Robert, C., Daud, A., Hodi, F. S., Hwu, W. J., Kefford, R., Wolchok, J. D., Hersey, P., Joseph, R. W., Weber, J. S., Dronca, R., Gangadhar, T. C., Patnaik, A., Zarour, H., Joshua, A. M., Gergich, K., Elassaiss-Schaap, J., Algazi, A., Mateus, C., Boasberg, P., Tumeh, P. C., Chmielowski, B., Ebbinghaus, S. W., LI, X. N., Kang, S. P., & Ribas, A. (2013). Safety and tumor responses with lambrolizumab (anti-PD-1) in melanoma. *The New England Journal of Medicine, 369*, 134–144.

Harrington, K. J., Ferris, R. L., Blumenschein, G., Jr., Colevas, A. D., Fayette, J., Licitra, L., Kasper, S., Even, C., Vokes, E. E., Worden, F., Saba, N. F., Kiyota, N., Haddad, R., Tahara, M., Grunwald, V., Shaw, J. W., Monga, M., Lynch, M., Taylor, F., Derosa, M., Morrissey, L., Cocks, K., Gillison, M. L., & Guigay, J. (2017). Nivolumab versus standard, single-agent therapy of investigator's choice in recurrent or metastatic squamous cell carcinoma of the head and neck (CheckMate 141): Health-related quality-of-life results from a randomised, phase 3 trial. *The Lancet Oncology, 18*, 1104–1115.

Hideshima, T., Bergsagel, P. L., Kuehl, W. M., & Anderson, K. C. (2004). Advances in biology of multiple myeloma: Clinical applications. *Blood, 104*, 607–618.

Higano, C. S., Schellhammer, P. F., Small, E. J., Burch, P. A., Nemunaitis, J., Yuh, L., Provost, N., & Frohlich, M. W. (2009). Integrated data from 2 randomized, double-blind, placebo-controlled, phase 3 trials of active cellular immunotherapy with sipuleucel-T in advanced prostate cancer. *Cancer, 115*, 3670–3679.

Hodi, F. S., O'day, S. J., Mcdermott, D. F., Weber, R. W., Sosman, J. A., Haanen, J. B., Gonzalez, R., Robert, C., Schadendorf, D., Hassel, J. C., Akerley, W., Van Den Eertwegh, A. J., Lutzky, J., Lorigan, P., Vaubel, J. M., Linette, G. P., Hogg, D., Ottensmeier, C. H., Lebbe, C., Peschel, C., Quirt, I., Clark, J. I., Wolchok, J. D., Weber, J. S., Tian, J., Yellin, M. J., Nichol, G. M., Hoos, A., & Urba, W. J. (2010). Improved survival with ipilimumab in patients with metastatic melanoma. *The New England Journal of Medicine, 363*, 711–723.

Hu, J. C., Coffin, R. S., Davis, C. J., Graham, N. J., Groves, N., Guest, P. J., Harrington, K. J., James, N. D., Love, C. A., Mcneish, I., Medley, L. C., Michael, A., Nutting, C. M., Pandha, H. S., Shorrock, C. A., Simpson, J., Steiner, J., Steven, N. M., Wright, D., & Coombes, R. C. (2006). A phase I study of OncoVEXGM-CSF, a second-generation oncolytic herpes simplex virus expressing granulocyte macrophage colony-stimulating factor. *Clinical Cancer Research, 12*, 6737–6747.

Ives, N. J., Stowe, R. L., Lorigan, P., & Wheatley, K. (2007). Chemotherapy compared with bio-chemotherapy for the treatment of metastatic melanoma: A meta-analysis of 18 trials involving 2,621 patients. *Journal of Clinical Oncology, 25*, 5426–5434.

Jiang, T., Zhou, C., & Ren, S. (2016). Role of IL-2 in cancer immunotherapy. *Oncoimmunology, 5*, e1163462.

Kantoff, P. W., Higano, C. S., Shore, N. D., Berger, E. R., Small, E. J., Penson, D. F., Redfern, C. H., Ferrari, A. C., Dreicer, R., Sims, R. B., Xu, Y., Frohlich, M. W., Schellhammer, P. F., & Investigators, I. S. (2010). Sipuleucel-T immunotherapy for castration-resistant prostate cancer. *The New England Journal of Medicine, 363*, 411–422.

Kaufman, H. L., & Bines, S. D. (2010). OPTIM trial: A Phase III trial of an oncolytic herpes virus encoding GM-CSF for unresectable stage III or IV melanoma. *Future Oncology, 6*, 941–949.

Kaufman, H. L., Kohlhapp, F. J., & Zloza, A. (2015). Oncolytic viruses: A new class of immunotherapy drugs. *Nature Reviews. Drug Discovery, 14*, 642–662.

Kirkwood, J. M., Ibrahim, J. G., Sosman, J. A., Sondak, V. K., Agarwala, S. S., Ernstoff, M. S., & Rao, U. (2001). High-dose interferon alfa-2b significantly prolongs relapse-free and overall survival compared with the GM2-KLH/QS-21 vaccine in patients with resected stage IIB-III melanoma: Results of intergroup trial E1694/S9512/C509801. *Journal of Clinical Oncology, 19*, 2370–2380.

Larkin, J., Minor, D., D'angelo, S., Neyns, B., Smylie, M., Miller, W. H. Jr., Gutzmer, R., Linette, G., Chmielowski, B., Lao, C. D., Lorigan, P., Grossmann, K., Hassel, J. C., Sznol, M., Daud, A., Sosman, J., Khushalani, N., Schadendorf, D., Hoeller, C., Walker, D., Kong, G., Horak, C., & Weber, J. 2017. Overall survival in patients with advanced melanoma who received nivolumab versus investigator's choice chemotherapy in CheckMate 037: A randomized, controlled, open-label phase III trial. *Journal of Clinical Oncology*, JCO2016718023.

Lee, S., & Margolin, K. (2011). Cytokines in cancer immunotherapy. *Cancers (Basel), 3*, 3856–3893.

Li, M., Liu, X., Zhou, Y., & Su, S. B. (2009). Interferon-lambdas: The modulators of antivirus, anti-tumor, and immune responses. *Journal of Leukocyte Biology, 86*, 23–32.

Linsley, P. S., Bradshaw, J., Greene, J., Peach, R., Bennett, K. L., & Mittler, R. S. (1996). Intracellular trafficking of CTLA-4 and focal localization towards sites of TCR engagement. *Immunity, 4*, 535–543.

Liu, B. L., Robinson, M., Han, Z. Q., Branston, R. H., English, C., REAY, P., Mcgrath, Y., Thomas, S. K., Thornton, M., Bullock, P., Love, C. A., & Coffin, R. S. (2003). ICP34.5 deleted herpes simplex virus with enhanced oncolytic, immune stimulating, and anti-tumour properties. *Gene Therapy, 10*, 292–303.

Long, G. V., Weber, J. S., Larkin, J., Atkinson, V., Grob, J. J., Schadendorf, D., Dummer, R., Robert, C., Marquez-Rodas, I., Mcneil, C., Schmidt, H., Briscoe, K., Baurain, J. F., Hodi, F. S. & Wolchok, J. D. (2017). Nivolumab for patients with advanced melanoma treated beyond progression: Analysis of 2 phase 3 clinical trials. *JAMA Oncology*.

Lonial, S., Kaufman, J., Reece, D., Mateos, M. V., Laubach, J., & Richardson, P. (2016). Update on elotuzumab, a novel anti-SLAMF7 monoclonal antibody for the treatment of multiple myeloma. *Expert Opinion on Biological Therapy, 16*, 1291–1301.

Magen, H., & Muchtar, E. (2016). Elotuzumab: The first approved monoclonal antibody for multiple myeloma treatment. *Therapeutic Advances in Hematology, 7*, 187–195.

Mahoney, K. M., Rennert, P. D., & Freeman, G. J. (2015). Combination cancer immunotherapy and new immunomodulatory targets. *Nature Reviews. Drug Discovery, 14*, 561–584.

Mcdermott, D. F., Regan, M. M., Clark, J. I., Flaherty, L. E., Weiss, G. R., Logan, T. F., Kirkwood, J. M., Gordon, M. S., Sosman, J. A., Ernstoff, M. S., Tretter, C. P., Urba, W. J., Smith, J. W., Margolin, K. A., Mier, J. W., Gollob, J. A., Dutcher, J. P., & Atkins, M. B. (2005). Randomized phase III trial of high-dose interleukin-2 versus subcutaneous interleukin-2 and interferon in patients with metastatic renal cell carcinoma. *Journal of Clinical Oncology, 23*, 133–141.

Mellman, I., Coukos, G., & Dranoff, G. (2011). Cancer immunotherapy comes of age. *Nature, 480*, 480–489.

Mocellin, S., Pasquali, S., Rossi, C. R., & Nitti, D. (2010). Interferon alpha adjuvant therapy in patients with high-risk melanoma: A systematic review and meta-analysis. *Journal of the National Cancer Institute, 102*, 493–501.

Morgan, D. A., Ruscetti, F. W., & Gallo, R. (1976). Selective in vitro growth of T lymphocytes from normal human bone marrows. *Science, 193*, 1007–1008.

Motz, G. T., & Coukos, G. (2013). Deciphering and reversing tumor immune suppression. *Immunity, 39*, 61–73.

Nour, N. M. (2009). Cervical cancer: A preventable death. *Review of Obstetrics and Gynecology, 2*, 240–244.

Overwijk, W. W., Theoret, M. R., & Restifo, N. P. (2000). The future of interleukin-2: Enhancing therapeutic anti-cancer vaccines. *The Cancer Journal from Scientific American, 6*(Suppl 1), S76–S80.

Palucka, K., & Banchereau, J. (2012). Cancer immunotherapy via dendritic cells. *Nature Reviews. Cancer, 12*, 265–277.

Pasquali, S., & Mocellin, S. (2010). The anti-cancer face of interferon alpha (IFN-alpha): From biology to clinical results, with a focus on melanoma. *Current Medicinal Chemistry, 17*, 3327–3336.

Peace, D. J., & Cheever, M. A. (1989). Toxicity and therapeutic efficacy of high-dose interleukin 2. In vivo infusion of antibody to NK-1.1 attenuates toxicity without compromising efficacy against murine leukemia. *The Journal of Experimental Medicine, 169*, 161–173.

Peggs, K. S., Quezada, S. A., Korman, A. J., & Allison, J. P. (2006). Principles and use of anti-CTLA4 antibody in human cancer immunotherapy. *Current Opinion in Immunology, 18*, 206–213.

Platanias, L. C. (2013). Interferons and their anti-tumor properties. *Journal of Interferon & Cytokine Research, 33*(4), 143.

Quesada, J. R., Hersh, E. M., Manning, J., Reuben, J., Keating, M., Schnipper, E., Itri, L., & Gutterman, J. U. (1986). Treatment of hairy cell leukemia with recombinant alpha-interferon. *Blood, 68*, 493–497.

Reck, M., Rodriguez-Abreu, D., Robinson, A. G., Hui, R., Csoszi, T., Fulop, A., Gottfried, M., Peled, N., Tafreshi, A., Cuffe, S., O'brien, M., Rao, S., Hotta, K., Leiby, M. A., Lubiniecki, G. M., Shentu, Y., Rangwala, R., Brahmer, J. R., & Investigators, K. (2016). Pembrolizumab versus chemotherapy for PD-L1-positive non-small-cell lung cancer. *The New England Journal of Medicine, 375*, 1823–1833.

Robert, C., Schachter, J., Long, G. V., Arance, A., Grob, J. J., Mortier, L., Daud, A., Carlino, M. S., Mcneil, C., Lotem, M., Larkin, J., Lorigan, P., Neyns, B., Blank, C. U., Hamid, O., Mateus, C., Shapira-Frommer, R., Kosh, M., Zhou, H., Ibrahim, N., Ebbinghaus, S., Ribas, A., & Investigators, K. (2015). Pembrolizumab versus ipilimumab in advanced melanoma. *The New England Journal of Medicine, 372*, 2521–2532.

Robert, C., Thomas, L., Bondarenko, I., O'day, S., Weber, J., Garbe, C., Lebbe, C., Baurain, J. F., Testori, A., Grob, J. J., Davidson, N., Richards, J., Maio, M., Hauschild, A., Miller, W. H., Jr., Gascon, P., Lotem, M., Harmankaya, K., Ibrahim, R., Francis, S., Chen, T. T., Humphrey, R., Hoos, A., & Wolchok, J. D. (2011). Ipilimumab plus dacarbazine for previously untreated metastatic melanoma. *The New England Journal of Medicine, 364*, 2517–2526.

Rosenberg, S. A. (2014). IL-2: The first effective immunotherapy for human cancer. *Journal of Immunology, 192*, 5451–5458.

Rosenberg, S. A., Lotze, M. T., Muul, L. M., Leitman, S., Chang, A. E., Ettinghausen, S. E., Matory, Y. L., Skibber, J. M., Shiloni, E., Vetto, J. T., et al. (1985). Observations on the systemic administration of autologous lymphokine-activated killer cells and recombinant interleukin-2 to patients with metastatic cancer. *The New England Journal of Medicine, 313*, 1485–1492.

Rosenberg, S. A., Yang, J. C., & Restifo, N. P. (2004). Cancer immunotherapy: Moving beyond current vaccines. *Nature Medicine, 10*, 909–915.

Sabado, R. L., & Bhardwaj, N. (2013). Dendritic cell immunotherapy. *Annals of the New York Academy of Sciences, 1284*, 31–45.

Sasse, A. D., Sasse, E. C., Clark, L. G., Ulloa, L., & Clark, O. A. (2007). Chemoimmunotherapy versus chemotherapy for metastatic malignant melanoma. *Cochrane Database of Systematic Reviews*, (1), CD005413.

Schuler, G. (2010). Dendritic cells in cancer immunotherapy. *European Journal of Immunology, 40*, 2123–2130.

Schwartzentruber, D. J., Lawson, D. H., Richards, J. M., Conry, R. M., Miller, D. M., Treisman, J., Gailani, F., Riley, L., Conlon, K., Pockaj, B., Kendra, K. L., White, R. L., Gonzalez, R., Kuzel, T. M., Curti, B., Leming, P. D., Whitman, E. D., Balkissoon, J., Reintgen, D. S., Kaufman, H., Marincola, F. M., Merino, M. J., Rosenberg, S. A., Choyke, P., Vena, D., & Hwu, P. (2011). gp100 peptide vaccine and interleukin-2 in patients with advanced melanoma. *The New England Journal of Medicine, 364*, 2119–2127.

Sharpe, A. H., Wherry, E. J., Ahmed, R., & Freeman, G. J. (2007). The function of programmed cell death 1 and its ligands in regulating autoimmunity and infection. *Nature Immunology, 8*, 239–245.

Siegel, R. L., Miller, K. D., & Jemal, A. (2015). Cancer statistics, 2015. *CA: a Cancer Journal for Clinicians, 65*, 5–29.

Smith, F. O., Downey, S. G., Klapper, J. A., Yang, J. C., Sherry, R. M., Royal, R. E., Kammula, U. S., Hughes, M. S., Restifo, N. P., Levy, C. L., White, D. E., Steinberg, S. M., & Rosenberg, S. A. (2008). Treatment of metastatic melanoma using interleukin-2 alone or in conjunction with vaccines. *Clinical Cancer Research, 14*, 5610–5618.

Smyth, M. J., Dunn, G. P., & Schreiber, R. D. (2006). Cancer immunosurveillance and immunoediting: The roles of immunity in suppressing tumor development and shaping tumor immunogenicity. *Advances in Immunology, 90*, 1–50.

Stein, B. L., & Tiu, R. V. (2013). Biological rationale and clinical use of interferon in the classical BCR-ABL-negative myeloproliferative neoplasms. *Journal of Interferon & Cytokine Research, 33*, 145–153.

Tesfay, M. Z., Kirk, A. C., Hadac, E. M., Griesmann, G. E., Federspiel, M. J., Barber, G. N., Henry, S. M., Peng, K. W., & Russell, S. J. (2013). PEGylation of vesicular stomatitis virus extends virus persistence in blood circulation of passively immunized mice. *Journal of Virology, 87*, 3752–3759.

Toda, M., Martuza, R. L., & Rabkin, S. D. (2000). Tumor growth inhibition by intratumoral inoculation of defective herpes simplex virus vectors expressing granulocyte-macrophage colony-stimulating factor. *Molecular Therapy, 2*, 324–329.

Tomita, Y., Fukasawa, S., Shinohara, N., Kitamura, H., Oya, M., Eto, M., Tanabe, K., Kimura, G., Yonese, J., Yao, M., Motzer, R. J., Uemura, H., Mchenry, M. B., Berghorn, E., & Ozono, S. (2017). Nivolumab versus everolimus in advanced renal cell carcinoma: Japanese subgroup analysis from the CheckMate 025 study. *Japanese Journal of Clinical Oncology*, 1–8.

Topalian, S. L., Weiner, G. J., & Pardoll, D. M. (2011). Cancer immunotherapy comes of age. *Journal of Clinical Oncology, 29*, 4828–4836.

Vansteenkiste, J., Betticher, D., Eberhardt, W., & De Leyn, P. (2007). Randomized controlled trial of resection versus radiotherapy after induction chemotherapy in stage IIIA-N2 non-small cell lung cancer. *Journal of Thoracic Oncology, 2*, 684–685.

Vedantham, S., Gamliel, H., & Golomb, H. M. (1992). Mechanism of interferon action in hairy cell leukemia: A model of effective cancer biotherapy. *Cancer Research, 52*, 1056–1066.

Veronese, F. M., & Mero, A. (2008). The impact of PEGylation on biological therapies. *BioDrugs, 22*, 315–329.

Yaddanapudi, K., Mitchell, R. A., & Eaton, J. W. (2013). Cancer vaccines: Looking to the future. *Oncoimmunology, 2*, e23403.

Chapter 3
Melanoma Immunotherapy

Matthew S. Block

Contents

Melanoma and the Immune System

Melanoma has long been considered one of the most "immunogenic" tumors. Early evidence suggesting that the host immune response could eradicate cancer came from observations that melanomas, including disseminated melanomas, would occasionally regress without therapy (Baker 1964; Everson 1967; Nathanson 1976). Although the mechanisms involved in spontaneous regression of melanoma were not initially known, many investigators felt that the host immune system was responsible. As the components of the cellular immune response were identified, a relationship was observed between tumor-infiltrating lymphocytes (TILs) and outcome in melanoma (Clark et al. 1969; Poppema et al. 1983; Strohal et al. 1994), and

M.S. Block (✉)
Department of Medical Oncology, Mayo Clinic, Rochester, MN, USA

© Springer International Publishing AG 2018   39
H. Dong, S.N. Markovic (eds.), *The Basics of Cancer Immunotherapy*,
https://doi.org/10.1007/978-3-319-70622-1_3

investigators noted a correlation between TILs and spontaneous melanoma regression (Mackensen et al. 1994). The demonstration that cloned TILs could recognize and lyse autologous melanoma cells provided an important proof of the concept of tumor immunotherapy (Topalian et al. 1989; Itoh et al. 1988; Sensi et al. 1993). This was further substantiated by the recognition that vitiligo (the loss of pigment in the skin due to destruction of benign melanocytes), which is seen in higher frequency in melanoma patients, is mediated by the immune system (Bystryn 1989). Because of the early recognition of the immunogenicity of melanomas (as well as the relative futility of cytotoxic chemotherapy and radiotherapy approaches to metastatic melanoma), melanoma has been the cancer in which immunotherapy has been most studied. Thus, to describe the rationale for various immunotherapies for melanoma, we will first discuss the means by which melanomas both stimulate and suppress the host anti-tumor immune response.

Inherent Immunogenicity of Melanoma

Once it became clear that the immune system was capable of recognizing melanomas, investigators sought to determine the antigens responsible for immune recognition. Melanoma antigens have been classified into cancer-testis antigens, overexpression antigens, melanocyte differentiation antigens, and neoantigens. Cancer-testis antigens are germline-encoded antigens with no expression or minimal expression by most tissues of the body, but are expressed in the testis (which normally has no HLA class I expression) and by a subset of melanoma cells. The prototypic cancer-testis antigens are the melanoma antigen-encoding (MAGE) proteins (Van Der Bruggen et al. 1991; Chomez et al. 2001). Overexpression antigens are normally expressed at low levels, but are expressed at higher levels by tumors; these include the proteins survivin (Schmitz et al. 2000), melanoma antigen preferentially expressed in tumors (PRAME) (Ikeda et al. 1997), and telomerase (Vonderheide et al. 1999). Melanocyte differentiation antigens have shared expression by melanoma cells and normal melanocytes. While the presence of differentiation antigens on non-malignant melanocytes suggests that self-tolerance may be a key concern, tumor-infiltrating lymphocytes recognizing the differentiation antigens Melan A (MART-1) (Kawakami et al. 1994), glycoprotein 100 (gp100) (Bakker et al. 1994), and tyrosinase (Brichard et al. 1993) have been described. Finally, with the advent of next-generation sequencing and algorithms capable of predicting the binding of peptide antigens to HLA molecules (Overwijk et al. 2013), antigens comprised of mutated proteins, referred to as neoantigens, have been shown to be recognized by a high proportion of melanoma TILs (Gros et al. 2016). Of note, because melanomas harbor a relatively high number of non-synonymous mutations, they have, on average, the highest number of neoantigens of any tumor type (Schumacher and Schreiber 2015).

In addition to being the tumor most capable of stimulating the adaptive immune response, melanoma stimulates the innate immune system via a variety of mechanisms.

Gene expression profiling of melanoma metastases has demonstrated significant expression of type I interferons IFNs) (Harlin et al. 2009), which are produced by innate immune cells in response to a variety of stimuli. Type I IFNs are typically produced in response to binding of a variety of innate immune receptors, including the toll-like receptors (TLRs), nod-like receptors (NLRs), C-type lectin receptors, and the STING receptor (Gajewski et al. 2012). Melanomas have been reported to express high levels of many damage-associated molecular patterns (DAMPs) capable of stimulating type I IFN production; this contributes to the inherent immunogenicity of melanoma.

Mechanisms of Immunosuppression Employed by Melanoma

Despite containing a relatively high number of antigens and innate immune stimuli, most advanced melanomas are not eradicated by the host immune response. This is due in part to immune editing (selection of subclones of melanoma cells that do not express dominant antigens), but is also due to melanoma-induced immunosuppression. Most melanoma immune-escape mechanisms involve alterations in the tumor microenvironment (TME). One key means of melanoma immune evasion is the loss of HLA class I molecules, leading to a lack of antigen presentation (Ferrone and Marincola 1995). Loss of class I molecules would be expected to lead to increased sensitivity to natural killer (NK) cell recognition and killing, but melanomas often downregulate NK cell ligands as well (Burke et al. 2010). In addition to the loss of ligands recognized by immune cells, melanomas elaborate many immunosuppressive factors into the TME, including vascular endothelial growth factor (VEGF), transforming growth factor beta (TGFβ), interleukin 10 (IL-10), and nitric oxide (NO) (Kusmartsev and Gabrilovich 2006). Many melanomas constitutively express indolamine 2,3-dioxygenase (IDO) enzymes, which convert tryptophan to kynurenine (Uyttenhove et al. 2003). Tryptophan is important for the function of cytotoxic T cells (CTL) and T-helper 1 (Th1) cells (Hwu et al. 2000), whereas kynurenine supports regulatory T cell (Treg) function (Mezrich et al. 2010). In this way, melanoma-mediated IDO expression leads to anergy of proinflammatory T cells and allows for an increase in immunosuppressive Tregs. Tregs, in turn, support expansion of myeloid-derived suppressor cells (MDSCs), which express arginase 1 (resulting in depletion of L-arginine, which is needed for effector T cell function) and inducible nitric oxide synthase (iNOS—resulting in the production of NO and reactive oxygen species) (Umansky and Sevko 2012).

Perhaps the most well-known immunosuppressive factor produced by melanoma is programmed death ligand 1 (PD-L1). By binding to the co-inhibitory receptor programmed death 1 (PD-1), PD-L1 activates tyrosine-protein phosphatase non-receptor type 11 (PTPN11, also known as Shp2) and decreases signaling through CD28 and the T-cell receptor. In most melanomas, PD-L1 is not constitutively expressed but is rather induced in response to one of several stimuli. Classically, PD-L1 expression is induced by IFN, which is expressed by TILs (Spranger et al. 2013). In this way, PD-L1 limits the degree of immune damage done to melanomas via upregulation in the context of Th1-mediated immune responses. Additionally, PD-L1 is upregulated in response to BRAF inhibition (Jiang et al. 2013), and thus can subvert the clinical efficacy of targeted therapy. While most investigators have focused on the immunosuppressive properties of membrane-bound PD-L1, a subset of melanomas also secrete a soluble splice variant of PD-L1 (Zhou et al. 2017); expression of soluble PD-L1 is a poor prognostic marker in melanoma. The key role played by PD-L1 in melanoma-mediated immunosuppression is perhaps best demonstrated by the clinical efficacy of antibodies that disrupt the interaction between PD-L1 and PD-1, as discussed below.

While the immunosuppressive mediators described above primarily work within the melanoma TME, melanomas have also been demonstrated to cause regional and systemic alterations in immunity, which can also lead to suppression of anti-melanoma immune responses. Sentinel lymph nodes from resected early-stage melanoma patients demonstrate evidence of Th2 polarization, including a decrease in CD8+ T cells and an increase in VEGF (Grotz et al. 2015). This repolarization of lymph nodes, which occurs even in stage I melanoma patients, is mediated in part through the elaboration of extracellular vesicles (EVs) (Maus et al. 2017), which contain several immunosuppressive factors. Once melanoma has metastasized, many patients demonstrate systemic Th2 polarization, as demonstrated by Th1 cell dysfunction and high levels of Th2 cytokines circulating in plasma (Nevala et al. 2009). Patients with metastatic melanoma also exhibit decreased circulating dendritic cells (DCs) and altered monocyte function (Chavan et al. 2014). While the mechanisms behind the systemic shift from Th1- to Th2-dominated immunity are not completely clear, one cause may be galectin 9, which is commonly found in the plasma of metastatic melanoma patients, and which converts immune responses from Th1 to Th2 (Enninga et al. 2016). The presence of regional and systemic immune dysregulation has the potential to impact the efficacy of melanoma immunotherapies (see Table 3.1).

Table 3.1 Melanoma antigens and immunomodulatory properties of melanoma

Immunogenic factors	Immunosuppressive factors
High level of T-cell antigens	Antigen loss
Cancer-testis antigens (MAGE family, NY-ESO-1, etc.)	Loss of HLA molecules
Overexpression antigens (survivin, PRAME, telomerase, etc.)	Loss of NK cell ligands
Melanocyte differentiation antigens (MART-1, tyrosinase, gp100, etc.)	Production of immunosuppressive cytokines
Neoantigens (highest number of any tumor type due to high burden of non-synonymous mutations)	VEGF
Strong stimulation of innate immune system	TGFβ
Heat shock proteins	IL-10
Other DAMPs	NO
	PD-L1
	IDO (supports Tregs, inhibits CTLs and Th1s)
	MDSCs
	Th2-biasing of regional LN
	Systemic T2 repolarization

Adjuvant Immunotherapy for Melanoma

Once a primary melanoma has been resected, the risk for recurrence depends on the site of the primary tumor, the depth of invasion, and the presence or absence of regional lymph node metastasis. For a thin cutaneous melanoma with no lymph node metastasis, the risk of distant melanoma metastasis is minimal, and no systemic therapy is recommended. However, for non-cutaneous melanomas, thick primary cutaneous melanomas, and melanomas with lymph node metastasis, the risk of recurrence after definitive surgery is relatively high. Whereas the majority of resected solid organ cancers can be treated effectively with cytotoxic chemotherapy, this approach has not proven beneficial in the adjuvant setting for melanoma. However, two immunotherapy approaches—IFN α and ipilimumab—are approved by the US Food and Drug Administration (FDA) for the treatment of stage III melanoma following surgical resection, and other immunotherapy approaches are being tested in the adjuvant setting.

Interferon Alfa

Interferons are proteins produced naturally by the body in response to several pathogens, most notably viruses. IFNα is secreted by leukocytes of the innate immune system and stimulates a number of host immune functions, including induction of fever via the hypothalamus (Wang et al. 2004), increased expression of MHC class I molecules (Schiavoni et al. 2013), increased T-cell co-stimulation (Snell et al. 2017), and direct impairment of tumor cell growth (Balmer 1985).

Based on these properties, investigators have tested recombinant IFNα as an adjuvant therapy in patients with resected high-risk melanoma. Multiple randomized clinical trials have been conducted testing both aqueous and pegylated forms of IFNα. A meta-analysis of 18 randomized clinical trials testing adjuvant IFNα in patients with stage II and stage III melanoma showed that adjuvant IFNα improves disease-free survival (hazard ratio (HR) 0.83, confidence interval (CI) 0.78–0.87) and, to a small extent, overall survival (HR 0.91, CI 0.85–0.97) (Mocellin et al. 2013). The number of melanoma patients that must be treated with IFNα to prevent one death is approximately 35. Similarly, a second meta-analysis combining results from trials testing several different forms and dosing schedules of IFNα showed that the use of adjuvant IFNα was associated with a modest improvement in event-free survival and overall survival, with an absolute 10-year event-free survival benefit of 2.5% and overall survival benefit of 2.6% (Ives et al. 2017).

Unfortunately, the use of adjuvant IFNα is associated with considerable toxicity in some patients. The most common toxicities are fatigue, depression, liver test abnormalities, pyrexia, headache, and myalgia. Toxicity rates vary among different formulations of IFNα, with high-dose treatment (20 million units/m^2 intravenously (IV) at various frequencies) being more toxic than intermediate dose treatment

Table 3.2 Toxicities associated with interferon (IFN) α

Toxicity	Pegylated IFNα	High-dose IFNα	Intermediate-dose IFNα	Low-dose IFNα
Fatigue	16%	21–25%	13–15%	1–6%
Liver function tests	11%	27–29%	4–5%	2–4%
Pyrexia	5%	10–35%	19–22%	<1%
Headache	4%	10–12%	6%	0%
Myalgia	5%	15–17%	8%	3%
Depression	7%	40%	10–12%	1–4%

(5–10 million units/m^2 IV), low-dose treatment (3 million units/m^2 IV), or pegylated IFNα (6 μg/kg subcutaneously once weekly). A table comparing the rate of severe (grade 3 or higher) toxicities is shown in Table 3.2 (Di Trolio et al. 2015).

Because of its marginal oncologic efficacy and significant toxicity, the use of adjuvant IFNα for high-risk resected melanoma remains somewhat controversial despite FDA approval.

Ipilimumab

The discovery that the inducible T-cell surface protein cytotoxic T-lymphocyte antigen 4 (CTLA-4) functions as a coinhibitory receptor led rapidly to the finding that targeting of CTLA-4 with monoclonal antibodies can lead to the enhancement of anti-tumor immune responses (Leach et al. 1996). This led to the testing and subsequent FDA approval of the CTLA-4-binding monoclonal antibody ipilimumab in the setting of metastatic melanoma, as is discussed in section "Immunotherapy for Metastatic Melanoma" of this chapter. Given the success of adjuvant ipilimumab in the metastatic setting, investigators queried whether ipilimumab could provide benefit to patients with resected stage III melanoma. To that end, a trial was conducted comparing adjuvant ipilimumab dosed at 10 mg/kg with a placebo in patients with resected with stage III cutaneous melanoma (with the caveat that for patients with stage IIIA melanoma, the metastatic nodal focus must be greater than 1 mm in maximal diameter) (Eggermont et al. 2015). Adjuvant ipilimumab was associated with improved recurrence-free survival (HR 0.75, median RFS 26.1 months versus 17.1 months) and was approved by the FDA on this basis. It was later demonstrated that ipilimumab was also associated with an improvement in overall survival when compared with placebo (HR 0.72, 5-year overall survival 65.4% vs. 54.4%) (Eggermont et al. 2016). A trial comparing ipilimumab with IFN and comparing ipilimumab at 10 mg/kg versus 3 mg/kg is currently underway (U.S. Intergroup E1609, NCT01274338).

Although the mechanism of action of ipilimumab is distinct from that of IFN, ipilimumab can also cause significant immune-related toxicity, generally thought to

Table 3.3 Toxicities associated with adjuvant ipilimumab

Event	Any grade	Grade 3	Grade 4	Grade 5
Any immune-related event	90.4%	35.9%	5.7%	1.1%
Cutaneous events	63.3%	4.2%	0%	0%
Diarrhea	41.2%	9.8%	0%	0%
Colitis	15.5%	6.8%	0.8%	0.6%
Hypophysitis	16.3%	4.2%	0.2%	0%
Increased liver enzymes	17.6%	3.0%	1.3%	0%

be mediated by T-cell responses against the host. Moreover, the frequency of toxicity seen in resected melanoma patients is considerably higher than for patients treated in the metastatic setting. This may be due in part to the difference in immune potential between patients with resected versus metastatic melanoma, but is likely largely due to the difference in the dose of ipilimumab approved for adjuvant versus metastatic use (10 mg/kg vs. 3 mg/kg). For patients treated with adjuvant ipilimumab, the most common severe toxicities include diarrhea/colitis, hepatitis, and hypophysitis. Table 3.3 showing select toxicities associated with adjuvant ipilimumab is shown below (Eggermont et al. 2016). Of the patients allocated to ipilimumab treatment, 52% discontinued therapy due to adverse events. Changes in health-related quality of life were observed between ipilimumab- and placebo-treated patients during the induction phase of treatment, especially related to diarrhea and insomnia, but these differences did not continue after the completion of induction (Coens et al. 2017).

Other Adjuvant Immunotherapy Treatments

Multiple additional immunotherapeutic approaches are currently being tested in the adjuvant setting for resected melanoma. The success of the PD-1-targeting monoclonal antibodies nivolumab and pembrolizumab in metastatic melanoma (as discussed in section "Immunotherapy for Metastatic Melanoma" of this chapter) has led to multiple trials testing these agents alone or in combination with other immune-modulating drugs. In addition, vaccines targeting specific melanoma antigens, vaccines comprised of autologous or allogeneic melanoma cells, and passive immunization with tumor-infiltrating lymphocytes (TILs) have been and are being tested in multiple trials in resected melanoma patients. Finally, other cytokines such as recombinant granulocyte-macrophage colony-stimulating factor (GM-CSF, sargramostim) have been tested (Lawson et al. 2015). While at present IFNα and ipilimumab are the only FDA-approved immunotherapy interventions for resected high-risk melanoma, it is likely that additional advances will be reported in the near future.

Immunotherapy for Metastatic Melanoma

Perhaps no other solid organ cancer setting has experienced a more dramatic clinical impact from immunotherapy than that of metastatic melanoma. While there is a longstanding history of the use of high-dose interleukin 2 and tumor-infiltrating lymphocytes in metastatic melanoma patients, the advent of immune checkpoint-inhibiting monoclonal antibodies has allowed immunotherapy to emerge as a standard-of-care for first-line therapy of metastatic melanoma. Whereas prior to the advent of immune checkpoint inhibitor therapy, the median overall survival of patients with metastatic melanoma was 6.2 months (Korn et al. 2008), many current clinical trials in metastatic melanoma demonstrate median survivals in excess of 2 years. While other drugs (namely small-molecule inhibitors of BRAF and MEK) have undoubtedly contributed to this increase in patients with BRAF-mutated melanoma, immunotherapies have been responsible for the majority of this improvement in clinical outcomes. In addition, melanoma is the first tumor for which an oncolytic virus has demonstrated clinical benefit in a randomized phase 3 clinical trial.

High-Dose Interleukin 2

Interleukin 2 (IL-2) is a cytokine produced by activated T cells. It serves as a growth factor for T cells and NK cells. Upon binding to its receptor, IL-2 activates multiple pathways within T and NK cells to drive cell proliferation and prevent apoptotic cell death. It is hypothesized that the basis for clinical benefit observed in select patients is that IL-2 drives expansion of melanoma-specific T cells and allows them to infiltrate tumors. However, the IL-2 receptor is also expressed by regulatory T cells (Tregs). Expansion of Tregs may be one reason why clinical benefit from IL-2 therapy is far from universal (Nicholas and Lesinski 2011).

Recombinant IL-2 therapy has been studied both as a single agent and in combination with IFN and with cytotoxic chemotherapy. A case record-based analysis of 631 patients treated on multiple clinical trials demonstrated a single-agent response rate of 14.9%, a response rate to IL-2 plus chemotherapy of 20.8%, a response rate to IL-2 plus IFN of 23.0%, and a response rate to IL-2 plus IFN plus chemotherapy (known as biochemotherapy) of 44.9% (Keilholz et al. 1998). The median overall survival for the entire cohort was 10.5 months; median survival times of patients treated with IL-2 alone, IL-2 plus chemotherapy, IL-2 plus IFN, and IL-2 plus IFN plus chemotherapy were 7.5, 9.9, 10.5, and 11.4 months, respectively.

Due to adverse events such as respiratory distress and capillary leak syndrome, IL-2 is often administered in the intensive care unit. The potential for severe adverse events has limited the use of high-dose IL-2 to specialized high-volume centers. Commonly observed grade 3 and higher toxicities include nausea, vomiting, hypotension, renal dysfunction, hepatic dysfunction, anemia requiring transfusion, thrombocytopenia, and neutropenic fever. In one meta-analysis, toxicity-related deaths occurred in 1.7% of patients (16/948) (Petrella et al. 2007).

Tumor-Infiltrating Lymphocyte (TIL) Therapy

Given the documented ability of T cells to recognize melanoma antigens and to lyse melanoma cells *in vitro*, investigators have been intrigued by the possibility of passively immunizing patients with melanoma-specific activated T cells. Since melanoma metastases frequently demonstrate T cell infiltrates; the concept of harvesting T cells from tumors (so-called tumor-infiltrating lymphocytes, or TILs), expanding them *in vitro* using cytokines, and re-infusing them into patients was developed. Initial trials of TILs rarely resulted in durable clinical benefit, as the TILs often failed to persist for more than a few days after adoptive transfer. However, the added steps of pre-conditioning patients with high doses of chemotherapy and infusing IL-2 after TIL therapy has led to improved TIL persistence and a higher frequency of objective responses, albeit at a cost of increased toxicity. For example, a trial of TIL therapy following intensive myeloablative chemotherapy led to objective responses in 49% of patients treated (the number of patients enrolled in the study was not reported, and so the intent-to-treat response rate cannot be calculated) (Dudley et al. 2008). Of patients treated, 56% had febrile neutropenia, 10% of patients required intubation, and 2% of patients died due to toxicity. Thus, while the objective response rate of TIL therapy is promising, the use of TILs has thus far been confined to a limited number of centers.

Ipilimumab

Whereas the unique toxicities and single patient manufacturing requirements of high-dose IL-2 and TIL therapies have limited their use to specialized institutions, the FDA approval of ipilimumab and its widespread adoption into clinical practice in 2011 ushered cancer immunotherapeutics into mainstream oncology. As discussed in section "Adjuvant Immunotherapy for Melanoma" of this chapter, ipilimumab binds to CTLA-4 and prevents it from binding to its ligands B7–1 and B7–2, thus preventing CTLA-4-driven coinhibitory signaling. As such, CTLA-4 blockade leads to increased expansion of activated T cells.

Ipilimumab was approved for use in metastatic melanoma on the basis of two randomized clinical trials. The first trial employed a 1:1:3 randomization of HLA-A2-positive previously treated metastatic melanoma patients to ipilimumab 3 mg/kg, a vaccine targeting gp100, or ipilimumab plus vaccine (Hodi et al. 2010). Although median progression-free survival was similar between the three groups, median overall survival was improved from 6.4 months in the vaccine-only arm to 10.1 and 10.0 months in the ipilimumab-only and ipilimumab plus vaccine arms, respectively. Importantly, the overall survival rates at 24 months were 23.5% and 21.6% for ipilimumab alone and ipilimumab plus vaccine, versus 13.7% for vaccine alone. The second trial randomized untreated metastatic melanoma patients to receive the cytotoxic chemotherapy drug dacarbazine (DTIC) plus placebo versus DTIC plus ipilimumab dosed at 10 mg/kg (Robert et al. 2011). Median overall survival was 9.1 months in the DTIC plus placebo arm and 11.2 months in the DTIC plus ipilimumab arm. Ultimately, the 3 mg/kg dose of ipilimumab was approved for use in metastatic melanoma.

Toxicities observed with ipilimumab are somewhat unique compared with those observed non-immune cancer therapeutics, in that the majority of toxicities are considered to be related to inflammatory responses targeting various organ systems. Immune-related toxicities include colitis, dermatitis, and hepatitis, among a host of others. In the above-mentioned clinical trials, grade 3 and 4 adverse events occurred in 45.8%, 45.5%, and 56.3% of patients treated with ipilimumab alone, ipilimumab plus vaccine, and ipilimumab plus DTIC, respectively. Most immune-related adverse events resolved with the use of steroids. However, management of immune-related toxicities remains a challenge in some patients, and toxicities that do not promptly resolve with steroid initiation should be managed by a multidisciplinary team (Kottschade et al. 2016).

Pembrolizumab and Nivolumab

Just as CTLA-4 is expressed on activated T cells as a co-inhibitory receptor to the B7–1 and B7–2 ligands, programmed death 1 (PD-1) is expressed by activated T cells and triggers T-cell death and anergy when bound by one of its ligands: PD-L1 (B7-H1) or PD-L2 (Dong and Chen 2003). PD-L1 is expressed by many tumors and tumor-infiltrating leukocytes; most often, PD-L1 expression is induced by IFNγ (Dong et al. 2002). In this way, expression of PD-L1 is a means for tumors to attenuate productive anti-tumor-immune responses.

Monoclonal antibodies that bind to PD-1 or PD-L1 can block the interaction between receptor and ligand and can prevent the resultant T-cell inhibition. In this way, anti-PD-1 antibodies allow for increased persistence of activated TILs in tumors that express PD-L1. The first PD-1-targeting monoclonal antibodies to be tested in clinical trials were pembrolizumab (initially known as lambrolizumab) and nivolumab.

The first report of pembrolizumab in melanoma was in 2013 by Dr. Hamid and colleagues (Hamid et al. 2013). Here, patients with advanced melanoma were treated with one of three dosing schedules: 10 mg/kg every 2 weeks, 10 mg/kg every 3 weeks, or 2 mg/kg every 3 weeks. Confirmed tumor responses were seen in 38% of patients, and responses rates were similar in patients who were naïve to ipilimumab or had received prior ipilimumab. On this basis, pembrolizumab at 2 mg/kg every 3 weeks was approved by the FDA for use in metastatic melanoma in patients who had previously been treated with ipilimumab.

Pembrolizumab was then compared with ipilimumab, which had emerged as a standard for first-line therapy of metastatic melanoma. Patients were randomized to receive either ipilimumab or pembrolizumab at 10 mg/kg every 2 weeks or pembrolizumab at 10 mg/kg every 3 weeks (Robert et al. 2015b). Median progression-free survival times were 5.5 months, 4.1 months, and 2.8 months for pembrolizumab every 2 weeks, pembrolizumab every 3 weeks, and ipilimumab, respectively.

Although median overall survival was not reached at the time of the trial report, the 12-month survival rates were 74.1%, 68.4%, and 58.2%, while the objective response rates were 33.7%, 32.9%, and 11.9% for pembrolizumab every 2 weeks, pembrolizumab every 3 weeks, and ipilimumab, respectively. On this basis, pembrolizumab was approved as first-line therapy for melanoma.

Similar to pembrolizumab, nivolumab is a monoclonal antibody that binds to PD-1 and disrupts the ability of PD-1 to bind to ligands and drive T-cell death and anergy. Nivolumab was developed in parallel as a single-agent therapy and in combination with ipilimumab. As a single agent, nivolumab was compared to DTIC in a placebo-controlled randomized phase III trial in untreated patients with metastatic melanoma without a BRAF mutation (Robert et al. 2015a). Here, nivolumab was given at 3 mg/kg every 2 weeks. Nivolumab therapy led to objective responses in 40.0% of patients, versus 13.9% of patients with DTIC. Median progression-free survival was 5.1 months with nivolumab versus 2.2 months with DTIC. Median overall survival was not reached for patients on nivolumab versus 10.8 months for patients on DTIC. Based on a significant improvement over DTIC, nivolumab was approved as monotherapy for metastatic melanoma.

The toxicities associated with single-agent pembrolizumab and single-agent nivolumab are similar both to each other and to those associated with ipilimumab. However, the frequency of severe adverse events was considerably lower for either anti-PD-1 therapy than for ipilimumab. Grade 3 or higher adverse events were seen in 34.8% of patients receiving pembrolizumab (Hamid et al. 2013) (31.8% of patients treated with 2 mg/kg every 3 weeks), and in 34% of patients treated with nivolumab (Robert et al. 2015a) (recall that 45.8% of patients treated with ipilimumab (Hodi et al. 2010) had grade 3 or higher adverse events). Thus, the PD-1-targeting drugs are associated with both higher objective response rates and lower toxicity as single agents than ipilimumab, which targets CTLA-4.

Combined Ipilimumab and Nivolumab

Given that CTLA-4 and PD-1 send distinct negative regulatory signals to T cells, and given that they are frequently engaged at different times and locations in the body, investigators hypothesized that combined targeting of CTLA-4 and PD-1 might lead to better control of melanoma than either agent alone. As such, the combination of ipilimumab (at 3 mg/kg every 3 weeks for four cycles) and nivolumab (1 mg/kg every 3 weeks for four cycles, followed by 3 mg/kg every 2 weeks) was compared against either agent alone in patients with untreated metastatic melanoma (Larkin et al. 2015). This led to statistical improvements in multiple oncologic outcomes over ipilimumab monotherapy, as well as numeric increases in multiple oncologic measures over nivolumab monotherapy. However, this improvement came at a cost of increased toxicity compared with either single agent. Nonetheless, the impressive rate of melanoma control by combined therapy with ipilimumab and nivolumab led to FDA approval of the combination in 2015. A summary of the outcomes of this phase III trial is shown in Table 3.4.

Table 3.4 Comparison of outcomes with combined ipilimumab and nivolumab, single-agent nivolumab, and single-agent ipilimumab

Regimen	Ipilimumab + nivolumab	Nivolumab	Ipilimumab
Objective response rate	57.6%	43.7%	19.0%
Median progression-free survival (months)	11.5	6.9	2.9
Grade 3+ adverse events	68.7%	43.5%	55.6%
Grade 3+ treatment-related adverse events	55.0%	16.3%	27.3%

Talimogene Laherparepvec

While ipilimumab, pembrolizumab, and nivolumab act by blocking immune-inhibitory signals, Talimogene Laherparepvec (T-VEC) is an oncolytic virus that, when injected intratumorally, stimulates the immune system both by directly killing tumor cells and by secreting the cytokine GM-CSF. GM-CSF serves as a chemoattractant for multiple leukocytes and recruits them into the tumor, where they encounter antigens released by killed melanoma cells, thus stimulating the anti-tumor immune response (Kohlhapp and Kaufman 2016).

Intratumoral T-VEC was compared against subcutaneously administered GM-CSF in patients with unresectable stage III or stage IV melanoma (Andtbacka et al. 2015). Overall response rate to T-VEC was 26.4% versus 5.7% for GM-CSF, while durable (> 6 months) response rate was 16.3% for T-VEC versus 2.1% for GM-CSF. The median overall survival for patients receiving T-VEC was 23.3 months versus 18.9 months for patients receiving GM-CSF. T-VEC was quite well tolerated, with cellulitis (2.1%) as the only severe adverse event occurring in more than 2% of patients. The trial was criticized due to the fact that GM-CSF is not considered by many to be a reasonable standard-of-care for patients with metastatic melanoma; however, T-VEC was approved by the FDA and is an active agent, particularly for patients with unresectable stage III and stage IVa melanoma (melanoma involving only subcutaneous sites and/or lymph nodes). T-VEC is generally not considered appropriate as monotherapy for patients with melanoma involving the lungs or other visceral organs; however, trials testing combinations of T-VEC with immune checkpoint inhibitors are ongoing.

Ongoing Clinical Trials

The success of anti-CTLA-4 and anti-PD-1 monoclonal antibodies for patients with metastatic melanoma has led to a multitude of clinical trials testing additional immunotherapies. These include blocking monoclonal antibodies to other immune checkpoints, immunostimulatory monoclonal antibodies, cytokines, vaccines, oncolytic viruses, and small-molecule inhibitors of proteins involved in modulating the nature of the immune response, as well as combinations of the above and combinations of immunotherapies with other treatments. It is beyond the scope of this book to discuss all of the ongoing clinical research efforts in the field of melanoma immunotherapy. However, it is worth mentioning the interesting clinical data regarding small molecule inhibitors of the IDO enzyme (see section "Melanoma and the Immune System" of this chapter), as these have shown intriguing clinical activity in combination with PD-1-blocking antibodies, with little added toxicity. Specifically, trials testing pembrolizumab combined with the IDO inhibitors epacadostat and indoximod have been reported in abstract form (Zakharia et al. 2016), and have noted objective responses in over 50% of patients with untreated metastatic melanoma with minimal increases in toxicity over pembrolizumab monotherapy. Randomized phase III trials testing these combinations are underway (NCT02752074 on www.clinicaltrials.gov).

Summary

In summary, melanomas tend to be quite immunogenic, but employ many mechanisms to evade or subvert anti-melanoma immune responses. At present, adjuvant ipilimumab is considered standard-of-care for patients with resected stage III melanoma. For patients with metastatic melanoma, patient outcomes have dramatically improved thanks in part to the use of ipilimumab, pembrolizumab, nivolumab, and T-VEC. With additional immunosuppressive pathways being targeted in ongoing clinical research, it is likely that additional immunotherapies for melanoma will prove useful in the near future.

Take Home Messages for Patients

- The role of the immune system in fighting melanoma has been long studied. Because of this relationship between immunity and melanoma, and because of the relative futility of chemotherapy and radiotherapy in treating metastatic melanoma, melanoma is the cancer in which immunotherapy has been most researched.
- Melanomas have been known to suppress the immune system through various mechanisms. One of the most classic ways is by expressing PD-L1, which binds to PD-1 expressed on the immune T cells, resulting in inactivation of the T cells.

Adjuvant (post-operative) immunotherapy in melanoma

- Whereas the majority of resected solid organ cancers can be treated effectively with chemotherapy, this approach has not proven beneficial in the adjuvant setting for melanoma. However, two immunotherapy approaches—IFNα and ipilimumab—are approved by the FDA for the treatment of stage III melanoma following surgical resection, and other immunotherapy approaches are being tested

- IFNs are proteins produced naturally by the body in response to several pathogens, most notably viruses. Investigators have tested recombinant IFNα as an adjuvant therapy in patients with resected high-risk melanoma. By collecting and analyzing the results of multiple trials, we have seen that adjuvant IFNα in patients with stage II and stage III melanoma can improve disease-free survival, and to a smaller extent, overall survival.
- Unfortunately, the use of adjuvant IFNα is associated with considerable side effects in some patients. The most common ones are fatigue, depression, liver test abnormalities, fever, headache, and muscle aches.
- T cells have an inhibitory protein on their surface called CTLA-4. By using the antibody ipilimumab to target CTLA-4, we can allow T cells to become more activated and induce stronger immune responses. This led to the testing and subsequent FDA approval of ipilimumab in the setting of metastatic melanoma as well as resected stage III melanoma.
- For patients treated with adjuvant ipilimumab, the most common severe toxicities include diarrhea, inflammation of the liver, and inflammation of the pituitary gland.

Immunotherapy in metastatic melanoma

- Interleukin 2 (IL-2) is a molecule produced by activated T cells that serves to activate T cells and other immune cells.
- IL-2 therapy has been studied both as a single agent and in combination with IFNα and with cytotoxic chemotherapy. A case record-based analysis of 631 patients treated on multiple clinical trials demonstrated a single-agent response rate of 14.9%, a response rate to IL-2 plus chemotherapy of 20.8%, a response rate to IL-2 plus IFNα of 23.0%, and a response rate to IL-2 plus IFNα plus chemotherapy of 44.9%.
- The potential for severe adverse events such as vomiting, shortness of breath, low blood pressure, kidney injury, liver injury, and blood disorders has limited the use of high-dose IL-2 to specialized high-volume centers.
- In 2011, the FDA approved the use of ipilimumab for metastatic melanoma based on the results of trials showing that adding ipilimumab to chemotherapy improved the survival of patients
- As mentioned earlier, expression of PD-L1 is a means for tumors to inhibit immune responses by binding to PD-1 on T cells and inactivating them. By using antibodies to block PD-1, we can restore the immune function and allow our immune cells to resume fighting the cancer. The first PD-1-targeting antibodies to be tested in clinical trials were pembrolizumab and nivolumab.
- Pembrolizumab was approved as first-line therapy for melanoma when it was shown to result in improved survival rates compared to ipilimumab.
- Nivolumab was approved as a single-agent option for metastatic melanoma when it was shown to result in improved survival rates compared to combined chemotherapy

- The side effects of pembrolizumab and nivolumab are similar in nature to ipilimumab (diarrhea, liver inflammation, skin rash), but occur at lower frequency than with ipilimumab.
- Combining ipilimumab with nivolumab was shown to result in even greater response rates and progression-free survival. However, this improvement came at a cost of increased toxicity compared with either single agent.
- While ipilimumab, pembrolizumab, and nivolumab act by blocking immune-inhibitory signals, Talimogene Laherparepvec (T-VEC) is a virus that when injected works by directly killing tumor cells and by secreting the molecule GM-CSF, which attracts immune cells to the tumor site. T-VEC is most helpful in controlling melanoma that has metastasized to skin, subcutaneous tissues, and/or lymph nodes.

References

Andtbacka, R. H., Kaufman, H. L., Collichio, F., Amatruda, T., Senzer, N., Chesney, J., Delman, K. A., Spitler, L. E., Puzanov, I., Agarwala, S. S., Milhem, M., Cranmer, L., Curti, B., Lewis, K., Ross, M., Guthrie, T., Linette, G. P., Daniels, G. A., Harrington, K., Middleton, M. R., Miller, W. H., Jr., Zager, J. S., Ye, Y., Yao, B., Li, A., Doleman, S., Vanderwalde, A., Gansert, J., & Coffin, R. S. (2015). Talimogene laherparepvec improves durable response rate in patients with advanced melanoma. *Journal of Clinical Oncology, 33*, 2780–2788.

Baker, H. W. (1964). Spontaneous regression of malignant melanoma. *The American Surgeon, 30*, 825–829.

Bakker, A. B., Schreurs, M. W., De Boer, A. J., Kawakami, Y., Rosenberg, S. A., Adema, G. J., & Figdor, C. G. (1994). Melanocyte lineage-specific antigen gp100 is recognized by melanoma-derived tumor-infiltrating lymphocytes. *The Journal of Experimental Medicine, 179*, 1005–1009.

Balmer, C. M. (1985). The new α interferons. *Drug Intelligence & Clinical Pharmacy, 19*, 887–893.

Brichard, V., Van Pel, A., Wolfel, T., Wolfel, C., De Plaen, E., Lethe, B., Coulie, P., & Boon, T. (1993). The tyrosinase gene codes for an antigen recognized by autologous cytolytic T lymphocytes on HLA-A2 melanomas. *The Journal of Experimental Medicine, 178*, 489–495.

Burke, S., Lakshmikanth, T., Colucci, F., & Carbone, E. (2010). New views on natural killer cell-based immunotherapy for melanoma treatment. *Trends in Immunology, 31*, 339–345.

Bystryn, J. C. (1989). Immune mechanisms in vitiligo. *Immunology Series, 46*, 447–473.

Chavan, R., Salvador, D., Gustafson, M. P., Dietz, A. B., Nevala, W., & Markovic, S. N. (2014). Untreated stage IV melanoma patients exhibit abnormal monocyte phenotypes and decreased functional capacity. *Cancer Immunology Research, 2*, 241–248.

Chomez, P., De Backer, O., Bertrand, M., De Plaen, E., Boon, T., & Lucas, S. (2001). An overview of the MAGE gene family with the identification of all human members of the family. *Cancer Research, 61*, 5544–5551.

Clark, W. H., Jr., From, L., Bernardino, E. A., & Mihm, M. C. (1969). The histogenesis and biologic behavior of primary human malignant melanomas of the skin. *Cancer Research, 29*, 705–727.

Coens, C., Suciu, S., Chiarion-Sileni, V., Grob, J. J., Dummer, R., Wolchok, J. D., Schmidt, H., Hamid, O., Robert, C., Ascierto, P. A., Richards, J. M., Lebbe, C., Ferraresi, V., Smylie, M., Weber, J. S., Maio, M., Bottomley, A., Kotapati, S., De Pril, V., Testori, A., & Eggermont, A. M. (2017). Health-related quality of life with adjuvant ipilimumab versus placebo after complete resection of high-risk stage III melanoma (EORTC 18071): Secondary outcomes of a multinational, randomised, double-blind, phase 3 trial. *The Lancet Oncology, 18*, 393–403.

Di Trolio, R., Simeone, E., Di Lorenzo, G., Buonerba, C., & Ascierto, P. A. (2015). The use of interferon in melanoma patients: A systematic review. *Cytokine & Growth Factor Reviews, 26*, 203–212.

Dong, H., & Chen, L. (2003). B7-H1 pathway and its role in the evasion of tumor immunity. *Journal of Molecular Medicine (Berl), 81*, 281–287.

Dong, H., Strome, S. E., Salomao, D. R., Tamura, H., Hirano, F., Flies, D. B., Roche, P. C., Lu, J., Zhu, G., Tamada, K., Lennon, V. A., Celis, E., & Chen, L. (2002). Tumor-associated B7-H1 promotes T-cell apoptosis: A potential mechanism of immune evasion. *Nature Medicine, 8*, 793–800.

Dudley, M. E., Yang, J. C., Sherry, R., Hughes, M. S., Royal, R., Kammula, U., Robbins, P. F., Huang, J., Citrin, D. E., Leitman, S. F., Wunderlich, J., Restifo, N. P., Thomasian, A., Downey, S. G., Smith, F. O., Klapper, J., Morton, K., Laurencot, C., White, D. E., & Rosenberg, S. A. (2008). Adoptive cell therapy for patients with metastatic melanoma: Evaluation of intensive myeloablative chemoradiation preparative regimens. *Journal of Clinical Oncology, 26*, 5233–5239.

Eggermont, A. M., Chiarion-Sileni, V., Grob, J. J., Dummer, R., Wolchok, J. D., Schmidt, H., Hamid, O., Robert, C., Ascierto, P. A., Richards, J. M., Lebbe, C., Ferraresi, V., Smylie, M., Weber, J. S., Maio, M., Bastholt, L., Mortier, L., Thomas, L., Tahir, S., Hauschild, A., Hassel, J. C., Hodi, F. S., Taitt, C., De Pril, V., De Schaetzen, G., Suciu, S., & Testori, A. (2016). Prolonged survival in stage III melanoma with ipilimumab adjuvant therapy. *The New England Journal of Medicine, 375*, 1845–1855.

Eggermont, A. M., Chiarion-Sileni, V., Grob, J. J., Dummer, R., Wolchok, J. D., Schmidt, H., Hamid, O., Robert, C., Ascierto, P. A., Richards, J. M., Lebbe, C., Ferraresi, V., Smylie, M., Weber, J. S., Maio, M., Konto, C., Hoos, A., De Pril, V., Gurunath, R. K., De Schaetzen, G., Suciu, S., & Testori, A. (2015). Adjuvant ipilimumab versus placebo after complete resection of high-risk stage III melanoma (EORTC 18071): A randomised, double-blind, phase 3 trial. *The Lancet Oncology, 16*, 522–530.

Enninga, E. A., Nevala, W. K., Holtan, S. G., Leontovich, A. A., & Markovic, S. N. (2016). Galectin-9 modulates immunity by promoting Th2/M2 differentiation and impacts survival in patients with metastatic melanoma. *Melanoma Research, 26*, 429–441.

Everson, T. C. (1967). Spontaneous regression of cancer. *Progress in Clinical Cancer, 3*, 79–95.

Ferrone, S., & Marincola, F. M. (1995). Loss of HLA class I antigens by melanoma cells: Molecular mechanisms, functional significance and clinical relevance. *Immunology Today, 16*, 487–494.

Gajewski, T. F., Fuertes, M. B., & Woo, S. R. (2012). Innate immune sensing of cancer: clues from an identified role for type I IFNs. *Cancer Immunology, Immunotherapy, 61*, 1343–1347.

Gros, A., Parkhurst, M. R., Tran, E., Pasetto, A., Robbins, P. F., Ilyas, S., Prickett, T. D., Gartner, J. J., Crystal, J. S., Roberts, I. M., Trebska-Mcgowan, K., Wunderlich, J. R., Yang, J. C., & Rosenberg, S. A. (2016). Prospective identification of neoantigen-specific lymphocytes in the peripheral blood of melanoma patients. *Nature Medicine, 22*, 433–438.

Grotz, T. E., Jakub, J. W., Mansfield, A. S., Goldenstein, R., Enninga, E. A., Nevala, W. K., Leontovich, A. A., & Markovic, S. N. (2015). Evidence of Th2 polarization of the sentinel lymph node (SLN) in melanoma. *Oncoimmunology, 4*, e1026504.

Hamid, O., Robert, C., Daud, A., Hodi, F. S., Hwu, W. J., Kefford, R., Wolchok, J. D., Hersey, P., Joseph, R. W., Weber, J. S., Dronca, R., Gangadhar, T. C., Patnaik, A., Zarour, H., Joshua, A. M., Gergich, K., Elassaiss-Schaap, J., Algazi, A., Mateus, C., Boasberg, P., Tumeh, P. C., Chmielowski, B., Ebbinghaus, S. W., Li, X. N., Kang, S. P., & Ribas, A. (2013). Safety and tumor responses with lambrolizumab (anti-PD-1) in melanoma. *The New England Journal of Medicine, 369*, 134–144.

Harlin, H., Meng, Y., Peterson, A. C., Zha, Y., Tretiakova, M., Slingluff, C., Mckee, M., & Gajewski, T. F. (2009). Chemokine expression in melanoma metastases associated with CD8+ T-cell recruitment. *Cancer Research, 69*, 3077–3085.

Hodi, F. S., O'day, S. J., Mcdermott, D. F., Weber, R. W., Sosman, J. A., Haanen, J. B., Gonzalez, R., Robert, C., Schadendorf, D., Hassel, J. C., Akerley, W., Van Den Eertwegh, A. J., Lutzky,

J., Lorigan, P., Vaubel, J. M., Linette, G. P., Hogg, D., Ottensmeier, C. H., Lebbe, C., Peschel, C., Quirt, I., Clark, J. I., Wolchok, J. D., Weber, J. S., Tian, J., Yellin, M. J., Nichol, G. M., Hoos, A., & Urba, W. J. (2010). Improved survival with ipilimumab in patients with metastatic melanoma. *The New England Journal of Medicine, 363*, 711–723.

Hwu, P., Du, M. X., Lapointe, R., Do, M., Taylor, M. W., & Young, H. A. (2000). Indoleamine 2,3-dioxygenase production by human dendritic cells results in the inhibition of T cell proliferation. *Journal of Immunology, 164*, 3596–3599.

Ikeda, H., Lethe, B., Lehmann, F., Van Baren, N., Baurain, J. F., De Smet, C., Chambost, H., Vitale, M., Moretta, A., Boon, T., & Coulie, P. G. (1997). Characterization of an antigen that is recognized on a melanoma showing partial HLA loss by CTL expressing an NK inhibitory receptor. *Immunity, 6*, 199–208.

Itoh, K., Platsoucas, C. D., & Balch, C. M. (1988). Autologous tumor-specific cytotoxic T lymphocytes in the infiltrate of human metastatic melanomas. Activation by interleukin 2 and autologous tumor cells, and involvement of the T cell receptor. *The Journal of Experimental Medicine, 168*, 1419–1441.

Ives, N. J., Suciu, S., Eggermont, A. M. M., Kirkwood, J., Lorigan, P., Markovic, S. N., Garbe, C., Wheatley, K., & International Melanoma Meta-Analysis Collaborative, G. (2017). Adjuvant interferon-α for the treatment of high-risk melanoma: An individual patient data meta-analysis. *European Journal of Cancer, 82*, 171–183.

Jiang, X., Zhou, J., Giobbie-Hurder, A., Wargo, J., & Hodi, F. S. (2013). The activation of MAPK in melanoma cells resistant to BRAF inhibition promotes PD-L1 expression that is reversible by MEK and PI3K inhibition. *Clinical Cancer Research, 19*, 598–609.

Kawakami, Y., Eliyahu, S., Sakaguchi, K., Robbins, P. F., Rivoltini, L., Yannelli, J. R., Appella, E., & Rosenberg, S. A. (1994). Identification of the immunodominant peptides of the MART-1 human melanoma antigen recognized by the majority of HLA-A2-restricted tumor infiltrating lymphocytes. *The Journal of Experimental Medicine, 180*, 347–352.

Keilholz, U., Conradt, C., Legha, S. S., Khayat, D., Scheibenbogen, C., Thatcher, N., Goey, S. H., Gore, M., Dorval, T., Hancock, B., Punt, C. J., Dummer, R., Avril, M. F., Brocker, E. B., Benhammouda, A., Eggermont, A. M., & Pritsch, M. (1998). Results of interleukin-2-based treatment in advanced melanoma: a case record-based analysis of 631 patients. *Journal of Clinical Oncology, 16*(9), 2921.

Kohlhapp, F. J., & Kaufman, H. L. (2016). Molecular pathways: Mechanism of action for talimogene laherparepvec, a new oncolytic virus immunotherapy. *Clinical Cancer Research, 22*, 1048–1054.

Korn, E. L., Liu, P. Y., Lee, S. J., Chapman, J. A., Niedzwiecki, D., Suman, V. J., Moon, J., Sondak, V. K., Atkins, M. B., Eisenhauer, E. A., Parulekar, W., Markovic, S. N., Saxman, S., & Kirkwood, J. M. (2008). Meta-analysis of phase II cooperative group trials in metastatic stage IV melanoma to determine progression-free and overall survival benchmarks for future phase II trials. *Journal of Clinical Oncology, 26*, 527–534.

Kottschade, L., Brys, A., Peikert, T., Ryder, M., Raffals, L., Brewer, J., Mosca, P., Markovic, S., & Midwest Melanoma, P. (2016). A multidisciplinary approach to toxicity management of modern immune checkpoint inhibitors in cancer therapy. *Melanoma Research, 26*, 469–480.

Kusmartsev, S., & Gabrilovich, D. I. (2006). Effect of tumor-derived cytokines and growth factors on differentiation and immune suppressive features of myeloid cells in cancer. *Cancer Metastasis Reviews, 25*, 323–331.

Larkin, J., Chiarion-Sileni, V., Gonzalez, R., Grob, J. J., Cowey, C. L., Lao, C. D., Schadendorf, D., Dummer, R., Smylie, M., Rutkowski, P., Ferrucci, P. F., Hill, A., Wagstaff, J., Carlino, M. S., Haanen, J. B., Maio, M., Marquez-Rodas, I., Mcarthur, G. A., Ascierto, P. A., Long, G. V., Callahan, M. K., Postow, M. A., Grossmann, K., Sznol, M., Dreno, B., Bastholt, L., Yang, A., Rollin, L. M., Horak, C., Hodi, F. S., & Wolchok, J. D. (2015). Combined nivolumab and ipilimumab or monotherapy in untreated melanoma. *The New England Journal of Medicine, 373*, 23–34.

Lawson, D. H., Lee, S., Zhao, F., Tarhini, A. A., Margolin, K. A., Ernstoff, M. S., Atkins, M. B., Cohen, G. I., Whiteside, T. L., Butterfield, L. H., & Kirkwood, J. M. (2015). Randomized, Placebo-Controlled, Phase III Trial of Yeast-Derived Granulocyte-Macrophage Colony-Stimulating Factor (GM-CSF) Versus Peptide Vaccination Versus GM-CSF Plus Peptide Vaccination Versus Placebo in Patients With No Evidence of Disease After Complete Surgical Resection of Locally Advanced and/or Stage IV Melanoma: A Trial of the Eastern Cooperative Oncology Group-American College of Radiology Imaging Network Cancer Research Group (E4697). *Journal of Clinical Oncology, 33*, 4066–4076.

Leach, D. R., Krummel, M. F., & Allison, J. P. (1996). Enhancement of anti-tumor immunity by CTLA-4 blockade. *Science, 271*, 1734–1736.

Mackensen, A., Carcelain, G., Viel, S., Raynal, M. C., Michalaki, H., Triebel, F., Bosq, J., & Hercend, T. (1994). Direct evidence to support the immunosurveillance concept in a human regressive melanoma. *The Journal of Clinical Investigation, 93*, 1397–1402.

Maus, R. L. G., Jakub, J. W., Nevala, W. K., Christensen, T. A., Noble-Orcutt, K., Sachs, Z., Hieken, T. J., & Markovic, S. N. (2017). Human melanoma-derived extracellular vesicles regulate dendritic cell maturation. *Frontiers in Immunology, 8*, 358.

Mezrich, J. D., Fechner, J. H., Zhang, X., Johnson, B. P., Burlingham, W. J., & Bradfield, C. A. (2010). An interaction between kynurenine and the aryl hydrocarbon receptor can generate regulatory T cells. *Journal of Immunology, 185*, 3190–3198.

Mocellin, S., Lens, M. B., Pasquali, S., Pilati, P., & Chiarion Sileni, V. (2013). Interferon α for the adjuvant treatment of cutaneous melanoma. *Cochrane Database of Systematic Reviews*, Cd008955.

Nathanson. (1976). Spontaneous regression of malignant melanoma: a review of the literature on incidence, clinical features, and possible mechanisms. *National Cancer Institute Monograph, 44*, 67–76.

Nevala, W. K., Vachon, C. M., Leontovich, A. A., Scott, C. G., Thompson, M. A., Markovic, S. N., & Melanoma Study Group Of The Mayo Clinic Cancer, C. (2009). Evidence of systemic Th2-driven chronic inflammation in patients with metastatic melanoma. *Clinical Cancer Research, 15*, 1931–1939.

Nicholas, C., & Lesinski, G. B. (2011). Immunomodulatory cytokines as therapeutic agents for melanoma. *Immunotherapy, 3*, 673–690.

Overwijk, W. W., Wang, E., Marincola, F. M., Rammensee, H. G., & Restifo, N. P. (2013). Mining the mutanome: Developing highly personalized Immunotherapies based on mutational analysis of tumors. *Journal of Immunotherapy Cancer, 1*, 11.

Petrella, T., Quirt, I., Verma, S., Haynes, A. E., Charette, M., Bak, K., & Melanoma Disease Site Group Of Cancer Care Ontario's Program In Evidence-Based, C. (2007). Single-agent interleukin-2 in the treatment of metastatic melanoma: A systematic review. *Cancer Treatment Reviews, 33*, 484–496.

Poppema, S., Brocker, E. B., De Leij, L., Terbrack, D., Visscher, T., Ter Haar, A., Macher, E., The, T. H., & Sorg, C. (1983). In situ analysis of the mononuclear cell infiltrate in primary malignant melanoma of the skin. *Clinical and Experimental Immunology, 51*, 77–82.

Robert, C., Long, G. V., Brady, B., Dutriaux, C., Maio, M., Mortier, L., Hassel, J. C., Rutkowski, P., Mcneil, C., Kalinka-Warzocha, E., Savage, K. J., Hernberg, M. M., Lebbe, C., Charles, J., Mihalcioiu, C., Chiarion-Sileni, V., Mauch, C., Cognetti, F., Arance, A., Schmidt, H., Schadendorf, D., Gogas, H., Lundgren-Eriksson, L., Horak, C., Sharkey, B., Waxman, I. M., Atkinson, V., & Ascierto, P. A. (2015a). Nivolumab in previously untreated melanoma without BRAF mutation. *The New England Journal of Medicine, 372*, 320–330.

Robert, C., Schachter, J., Long, G. V., Arance, A., Grob, J. J., Mortier, L., Daud, A., Carlino, M. S., Mcneil, C., Lotem, M., Larkin, J., Lorigan, P., Neyns, B., Blank, C. U., Hamid, O., Mateus, C., Shapira-Frommer, R., Kosh, M., Zhou, H., Ibrahim, N., Ebbinghaus, S., Ribas, A., & Investigators, K. (2015b). Pembrolizumab versus Ipilimumab in Advanced Melanoma. *The New England Journal of Medicine, 372*, 2521–2532.

Robert, C., Thomas, L., Bondarenko, I., O'day, S., Weber, J., Garbe, C., Lebbe, C., Baurain, J. F., Testori, A., Grob, J. J., Davidson, N., Richards, J., Maio, M., Hauschild, A., Miller, W. H., Jr., Gascon, P., Lotem, M., Harmankaya, K., Ibrahim, R., Francis, S., Chen, T. T., Humphrey, R., Hoos, A., & Wolchok, J. D. (2011). Ipilimumab plus dacarbazine for previously untreated metastatic melanoma. *The New England Journal of Medicine, 364*, 2517–2526.

Schiavoni, G., Mattei, F., & Gabriele, L. (2013). Type I interferons as stimulators of DC-mediated cross-priming: Impact on anti-tumor response. *Frontiers in Immunology, 4*, 483.

Schmitz, M., Diestelkoetter, P., Weigle, B., Schmachtenberg, F., Stevanovic, S., Ockert, D., Rammensee, H. G., & Rieber, E. P. (2000). Generation of survivin-specific CD8+ T effector cells by dendritic cells pulsed with protein or selected peptides. *Cancer Research, 60*, 4845–4849.

Schumacher, T. N., & Schreiber, R. D. (2015). Neoantigens in cancer immunotherapy. *Science, 348*, 69–74.

Sensi, M., Salvi, S., Castelli, C., Maccalli, C., Mazzocchi, A., Mortarini, R., Nicolini, G., Herlyn, M., Parmiani, G., & Anichini, A. (1993). T cell receptor (TCR) structure of autologous melanoma-reactive cytotoxic T lymphocyte (CTL) clones: tumor-infiltrating lymphocytes overexpress in vivo the TCR beta chain sequence used by an HLA-A2-restricted and melanocyte-lineage-specific CTL clone. *The Journal of Experimental Medicine, 178*, 1231–1246.

Snell, L. M., Mcgaha, T. L., & Brooks, D. G. (2017). Type I interferon in chronic virus infection and cancer. *Trends in Immunology, 38*, 542–557.

Spranger, S., Spaapen, R. M., Zha, Y., Williams, J., Meng, Y., Ha, T. T., & Gajewski, T. F. (2013). Up-regulation of PD-L1, IDO, and T(regs) in the melanoma tumor microenvironment is driven by CD8(+) T cells. *Science Translational Medicine, 5*, 200ra116.

Strohal, R., Marberger, K., Pehamberger, H., & Stingl, G. (1994). Immunohistological analysis of anti-melanoma host responses. *Archives of Dermatological Research, 287*, 28–35.

Topalian, S. L., Solomon, D., & Rosenberg, S. A. (1989). Tumor-specific cytolysis by lymphocytes infiltrating human melanomas. *Journal of Immunology, 142*, 3714–3725.

Umansky, V., & Sevko, A. (2012). Melanoma-induced immunosuppression and its neutralization. *Seminars in Cancer Biology, 22*, 319–326.

Uyttenhove, C., Pilotte, L., Theate, I., Stroobant, V., Colau, D., Parmentier, N., Boon, T., & Van Den Eynde, B. J. (2003). Evidence for a tumoral immune resistance mechanism based on tryptophan degradation by indoleamine 2,3-dioxygenase. *Nature Medicine, 9*, 1269–1274.

Van Der Bruggen, P., Traversari, C., Chomez, P., Lurquin, C., De Plaen, E., Van Den Eynde, B., Knuth, A., & Boon, T. (1991). A gene encoding an antigen recognized by cytolytic T lymphocytes on a human melanoma. *Science, 254*, 1643–1647.

Vonderheide, R. H., Hahn, W. C., Schultze, J. L., & Nadler, L. M. (1999). The telomerase catalytic subunit is a widely expressed tumor-associated antigen recognized by cytotoxic T lymphocytes. *Immunity, 10*, 673–679.

Wang, Y. X., Xu, W. G., Sun, X. J., Chen, Y. Z., Liu, X. Y., Tang, H., & Jiang, C. L. (2004). Fever of recombinant human interferon-α is mediated by opioid domain interaction with opioid receptor inducing prostaglandin E2. *Journal of Neuroimmunology, 156*, 107–112.

Zakharia, Y., Drabick, J. J., Khleif, S., Mcwilliams, R. R., Munn, D., Link, C. J., Vahanian, N. N., Kennedy, E., Shaheen, M. F., Rixe, O., & Milhem, M. M. (2016). Updates on phase1b/2 trial of the indoleamine 2,3-dioxygenase pathway (IDO) inhibitor indoximod plus checkpoint inhibitors for the treatment of unresectable stage 3 or 4 melanoma. *Journal of Clinical Oncology, 34*.

Zhou, J., Mahoney, K. M., Giobbie-Hurder, A., Zhao, F., Lee, S., Liao, X., Rodig, S., Li, J., Wu, X., Butterfield, L. H., Piesche, M., Manos, M. P., Eastman, L. M., Dranoff, G., Freeman, G. J., & Hodi, F. S. (2017). Soluble PD-L1 as a biomarker in malignant melanoma treated with checkpoint blockade. *Cancer Immunology Research, 5*, 480–492.

Chapter 4
Significance of Immune Checkpoints in Lung Cancer

Konstantinos Leventakos and Aaron S. Mansfield

Contents

Introduction

Lung cancer is the most common cause of cancer-related mortality in the USA (Siegel et al. 2017) and worldwide (Ferlay et al. 2015). As such, lung cancer represents a major global disease burden. Over the last few years there have been major advances in the treatment of lung cancer with the development of drugs that can target specific molecular abnormalities and with the advent of immunotherapy.

Lung cancer is not a single disease but it represents many types of cancers that can arise within the lungs. Lung cancer is classified primarily by whether it is small-cell lung cancer (SCLC) or non-small-cell lung cancer (NSCLC). There are multiple types of NSCLC but the two most common are adenocarcinoma and squamous cell carcinoma, of which adenocarcinoma is the most common. Sadly, many cases

K. Leventakos • A.S. Mansfield (✉)
Mayo Clinic, Division of Medical Oncology, Rochester, MN, USA

© Springer International Publishing AG 2018
H. Dong, S.N. Markovic (eds.), *The Basics of Cancer Immunotherapy*,
https://doi.org/10.1007/978-3-319-70622-1_4

of lung cancer are due to tobacco exposure, but a large proportion of these patients are never smokers. Other risk factors include radiation, asbestos, radon, and other environmental pollutants.

Staging and Treatments

The staging of lung cancer is very important because the stage of the cancer determines treatment options and influences survival. Although both NSCLC and SCLC are staged by the same TNM system, clinical decisions for SCLC are based on the Veterans Administration (VA) staging system. For NSCLCs that are localized to the lung, and whose removal would not significantly compromise pulmonary function, surgical removal of the tumor is considered. Sometimes because of co-morbidities such as cardiac or pulmonary disease, patients cannot undergo surgery, and ablation or radiotherapy may be considered instead. In patients with NSCLC that has spread to the lymph nodes in the mediastinum, consideration is given to a combination of cytotoxic chemotherapy and radiation therapy. In select cases with mediastinal involvement, patients may be considered for surgery. Once the disease has spread beyond the lung(s) and mediastinal lymph nodes, or if radiation therapy cannot be safely administered, systemic therapies are considered. Systemic treatment options can include cytotoxic chemotherapy, immunotherapy, or targeted therapy. The selection of targeted therapy depends on the detection of a mutation in *EGFR*, *ALK*, *ROS1*, or *BRAF* (Ettinger et al. 2017).

The treatment of SCLC is different to that of NSCLC. Surgery is rarely considered for SCLC. More commonly, if the diagnosis of SCLC is made, consideration for chemotherapy with radiation therapy is given if the disease is limited to a radiation port. If the disease is more widespread, chemotherapy alone is given with consideration of radiation to the chest or head afterwords, if not used previously. Immunotherapy is not yet FDA-approved for SCLC but is increasingly used based on recommendations from the National Comprehensive Cancer Network.

Immunotherapy

The treatment landscape of NSCLC is rapidly changing. The discovery of programmed cell death ligand 1 (PD-L1, aka B7-H1 and CD274) at the Mayo Clinic (Dong et al. 1999), the detection of PD-L1 on lung cancer tumor cells (Boland et al. 2013; Velcheti et al. 2014), and the negative regulation of T-cell proliferation through apoptosis of tumor-specific T-cells following engagement of PD-L1 with its receptor programmed cell death protein 1 (PD-1) (Dong et al. 2002), suggest that blocking the PD-L1/PD-1 axis in lung cancer is a reasonable therapeutic strategy for this malignancy (Pardoll 2012). As of 2017, three drugs that block this axis have been approved, and others are far along in development (Leventakos and Mansfield 2014, 2016).

Nivolumab

Nivolumab, a human IgG4 antibody that targets PD-1, was the first immunotherapy to receive approval for NSCLC in the USA. In a phase 1 dose-escalation cohort expansion trial, 129 patients with advanced NSCLC who had been receiving prior lines of therapy were included (Gettinger et al. 2015). The patients were almost equally distributed between squamous and non-squamous histologies. Subjects received nivolumab at 1, 3, or 10 mg/kg intravenously once every 2 weeks in 8-week cycles for up to 96 weeks. In the subjects receiving nivolumab 3 mg/kg, the median overall survival was 14.9 months (95% CI 7.3–30.3). The median overall survival was 9.2 months in both the 1- and 10-mg/kg cohorts. Overall response rates (ORR, the combination of complete and partial responses) were similar in subjects with squamous (16.7%) and non-squamous NSCLC (17.6%). Eighteen responding subjects discontinued nivolumab for reasons other than progressive disease; nine (50%) of those had responses that lasted more than 9 months after their last dose. Grade 3–4 treatment-related adverse events occurred in 14% of patients, of which fatigue (3.1%) and pneumonitis (2.3%) were most common. There were three treatment-related deaths associated with pneumonitis. Overall, this study determined the dose of nivolumab that was used in subsequent studies (3 mg/kg) and showed that nivolumab results in durable responses with encouraging survival rates in pre-treated patients with metastatic NSCLC.

CheckMate 063 restricted treatment to patients with squamous cell carcinoma (Rizvi et al. 2015b). In this phase 2 single-arm trial the therapeutic activity of nivolumab was tested in patients with advanced and refractory squamous NSCLC in Europe and the USA. The primary endpoint of this study was a confirmed ORR, and 17 of 117 subjects (14.5%) achieved a response. Whereas delayed responses with immune checkpoint inhibitors have been observed, the median time to response was 3.3 months. The majority of responses were still ongoing at the time of the report of this trial, and the median duration of responses still has not been published. In addition to the subjects who responded to treatment, 30 of 117 patients (26%) had stable disease (median duration 6 months, 95% CI 4.7–10.9 months). In this trial, there were two treatment-associated deaths (one due to pneumonia and one due to stroke) and grade 3–4 treatment related adverse events were present in 17% of subjects with fatigue (4%), pneumonitis (3%), and diarrhea (3%) being the most common. For 76 patients in this study, assessment of their pretreatment archival tumor samples for PD-L1 expression was possible. Using a cut-off of 5% expression of PD-L1 by tumor cells, 25 of 76 patients (33%) had positive tumors. Of the 25 patients with PD-L1-positive tumors and evaluable treatment responses, six of them (24%) achieved a partial response compared to 7 of 51 patients (14%) with PD-L1-negative tumors. This non-randomized, open-label clinical trial provided strong evidence that nivolumab is effective for the treatment of advanced and treatment-refractory squamous NSCLC. Furthermore, the data suggest that responses are independent of detectable PD-L1 expression in squamous NSCLC.

Subsequent to Checkmate 063, nivolumab was compared to docetaxel in a phase 3 randomized, open label, international clinical trial called CheckMate 017 for patients with squamous NSCLC (Brahmer et al. 2015). In this study, 272 patients were randomized to either treatment. Median overall survival was better with nivolumab (9.2 months, 95% CI 7.3–13.3) than with docetaxel (6.0 months, 95% CI 5.1–7.3). Similar to the phase 1 study and Checkmate 063, the response rate to nivolumab was 20%, which was significantly higher than that seen with docetaxel (9%). Progression-free survival was also significantly better for nivolumab (3.5 months) than for docetaxel (2.8 months). The two treatment groups were balanced for PD-L1 expression but this was neither prognostic nor predictive of benefit from nivolumab. Treatment-related grade 3 or 4 adverse events were more common with docetaxel (55%) and were attributable mainly to hematologic toxic events and infections. In comparison, only 7% of subjects who received nivolumab experienced grade 3 or 4 treatment-related adverse events, with the most common being fatigue, decreased appetite, and leukopenia.

CheckMate 017 confirmed that nivolumab provides meaningful survival benefit to patients with advanced, previously treated squamous-cell NSCLC with an improved safety profile compared to the standard-of-care. Nivolumab was approved by the US Food and Drug Administration (FDA) for patients with metastatic squamous NSCLC who have experienced progression with or after platinum-based chemotherapy based on data from CheckMate 063. The FDA approval did not make any statement about PD-L1 testing for patients with squamous NSCLC.

After the positive results of nivolumab in squamous NSCLC, this agent was compared to docetaxel in patients with non-squamous NSCLC that had progressed during or after platinum-based doublet chemotherapy in CheckMate 057 (Borghaei et al. 2015). The median overall survival was significantly better among the 292 subjects in the nivolumab group (12.2 months, 95% CI 9.7–15) than with the 290 subjects in the docetaxel group (9.4 months, 95% CI 8.1–10.7). Surprisingly, median progression-free survival was shorter in subjects who received nivolumab (2.3 months) than those who received docetaxel (4.2 months); however, the rate of progression-free survival at 1 year was higher with nivolumab (19%) than docetaxel (8%). The majority of subjects (78%) had tissue available for analysis of PD-L1 expression and rates of PD-L1 expression were balanced between the two treatment groups. In contrast with CheckMate 017 in squamous NSCLC where PD-L1 expression was not predictive of benefit, in this study PD-L1 expression in non-squamous NSCLC was strongly predictive of treatment benefit with nivolumab. Among subjects whose tumors expressed PD-L1, nivolumab nearly doubled the median overall survival as compared with those who received docetaxel. The hazard ratios in the analysis of overall survival did not favor nivolumab for the 82 patients with EGFR mutations, but definite conclusions are difficult due to the width of the confidence intervals (CI 0.69–2.00). Treatment-related grade 3 or 4 adverse events were reported in 10% of the patients in the nivolumab group, with fatigue, nausea, and diarrhea being the most common, as compared with 54% of those in the docetaxel group that experienced hematologic and infectious complications.

In CheckMate 057, this randomized, open-label, international phase 3 study showed the strong clinical benefit of nivolumab in patients with non-squamous NSCLC and the predictive role of PD-L1 expression for these patients. These results led to the extension of the FDA approval of nivolumab to non-squamous histology. The FDA also approved a complementary test for PD-L1 by immunohistochemistry (28–8 pharmDx) to guide physicians in patient selection for nivolumab treatment but a positive result is not needed for initiation of treatment.

Nivolumab has been tested as a single-agent for first-line treatment of NSCLC. In CheckMate 026, patients were randomized 1:1 to receive nivolumab or platinum-based chemotherapy (Carbone et al. 2017). Although patients with ≥ 1% PD-L1 tumor cell expression were included, the primary endpoint of progression-free survival as determined by independent central review was assessed only amongst patients with ≥ 5% PD-L1 tumor cell expression. Amongst 423 patients who were randomized with ≥ 5% PD-L1 tumor cell expression, median progression-free survival was 4.2 months for patients treated with nivolumab and 5.9 months for patients treated with chemotherapy (HR 1.15, 95% CI 0.91–1.45; p=0.25). overall survival was also similar between the groups, with a median of 14.4 months and 13.2 months for nivolumab and chemotherapy, respectively (HR 1.02, 95% CI 0.80–1.30). Crossover was allowed and 60% of patients initially treated with chemotherapy received subsequent nivolumab. As an exploratory endpoint, tumor-mutation burden was determined and patients were stratified based on this result. Patients with a high tumor mutation burden treated with nivolumab had a superior median progression-free survival (9.7 months) to those treated with chemotherapy (5.8 months; HR 0.62, 95% CI 0.38–1.0). In contrast, patients with low or medium tumor-mutation burdens treated with nivolumab had worse median progression-free survival (4.1 months) than those who received chemotherapy (6.9 months, HR 1.82, 95% CI 1.30–2.55). In summary, nivolumab is not superior to chemotherapy for frontline treatment of NSCLC when ≥ 5% PD-L1 tumor cell expression is used for selection. Nivolumab has not been approved for frontline treatment of NSCLC. Tumor mutation burden is a potential predictor of benefit to nivolumab such that patients with the highest burden may benefit the most, but validation is needed.

Pembrolizumab

The side effects, safety, and anti-tumor activity of pembrolizumab were first evaluated in a large phase 1, open-label clinical trial with 495 subjects with adenocarcinoma or squamous cell NSCLC at a ratio of approximately 4:1 (Garon et al. 2015). Most of the patients (81%) had received at least one previous treatment. Pembrolizumab was given at a dose of either 2 or 10 mg/kg every 3 weeks or 10 mg/kg every 2 weeks. Median overall survival was 12.0 months (95% CI 9.3–4.7) for all subjects, 9.3 months for previously-treated subjects, and 6.2 months for previously untreated subjects. The objective response rate was 19.4% with a median duration of response of 12.5 months for all of the subjects. In this study, 23.2% of subjects had detectable PD-L1 expression in at least 50% of tumor cells, and 37.6% of subjects had at least 1–49% of PD-L1 expression by tumor cells using the anti-PD-L1 antibody clone 22C3 (pharmDX). The median overall survival of the subjects with at least 50% tumor cell expression of PD-L1 was not reached (95% CI 13.7 months to not reached). Progression-free and overall survivals were higher for these subjects than other groups of expression. The most common side effects associated with pembrolizumab were fatigue, pruritus, and decreased appetite, regardless of dose or schedule. Almost 10% (47/495) of subjects experienced adverse events of grade 3 or higher, with the most common being dyspnea (3.8%) and pneumonitis (1.8%). Overall, this study suggested that pembrolizumab is effective and tolerable in patients with NSCLC. Clearly, PD-L1 expression was predictive of benefit with pembrolizumab; however, many more subjects were found to have any expression of PD-L1 with this clone than had been previously reported in NSCLC.

Based on the promising results of KEYNOTE-001, pembrolizumab was tested in an international, randomized, controlled, open-label, phase 2/3 study (KEYNOTE-010) (Herbst et al. 2016). Subjects with previously treated NSCLC with PD-L1 expression on at least 1% of tumor cells were randomly assigned 1:1:1 to receive pembrolizumab 2 mg/kg, pembrolizumab 10 mg/kg, or docetaxel every 3 weeks. Median overall survival was significantly longer for the subjects who received pembrolizumab: 10.4 months (95% CI 9.4–11.9) for the pembrolizumab 2 mg/kg group, 12.7 months (95% CI 10–17.3) for the pembrolizumab 10 mg/kg group, and 8.5 months (95% CI 7.5–9.8) for the docetaxel group. Median progression-free survival was almost equal for the three groups around 4 months. PD-L1 expression of at least 50% by tumor cells was predictive of improved survival with pembrolizumab than docetaxel, with median overall survival of 14.9 and 17.3 months for the groups of subjects treated with pembrolizumab 2 and 10 mg/kg, respectively, compared with subjects treated with docetaxel (8.2 months). During this trial, both archival and new tumor specimens were analyzed for PD-L1 expression, and detection from either was predictive of survival benefit with pembrolizumab. The subgroup analysis of overall survival suggested that there was benefit for subjects with adenocarcinoma (hazard ratio (HR) 0.63; 95% CI 0.5–0.79) and those with squamous NSCLC (HR 0.74; 95% CI 0.5–1.09). In accordance with what was observed in CheckMate 057 in patients with EGFR mutations, there was a trend for better outcomes with docetaxel treatment (HR 1.79; 95% CI 0.94–3.42), but the few patients with EGFR mutations who were included in this study limit any definite conclusions. Grade 3–5 treatment-related adverse events were less common with pembrolizumab than with docetaxel (13% of subjects who received 2 mg/kg, 16% of subjects who received 10 mg/kg, compared with 35% of subjects who received docetaxel). The most common grade 3–5 adverse event was pneumonitis (2%) in both of the pembrolizumab groups. Overall, KEYNOTE 010 demonstrated that pembrolizumab is relatively well tolerated and effective in patients with previously treated NSCLC whose tumors express PD-L1. Based on this study, the FDA granted accelerated approval for pembrolizumab in the treatment of patients with advanced NSCLC whose disease has progressed on or after other first-line therapies. The 22C3 clone for PD-L1 detection by IHC was also approved as a companion diagnostic test to identify tumors with PD-L1 expression. In contrast to nivolumab, a positive test for PD-L1 expression is needed for use of pembrolizumab.

Frontline Pembrolizumab

As of 2017 pembrolizumab is the only approved frontline PD-1 inhibitor for NSCLC. In the clinical trial that lead to this approval of pembrolizumab, patients with 50% or greater expression of PD-L1 on their tumor cells as detected by the 22C3 clone were randomized to receive pembrolizumab or the investigator's choice of standard-of-care chemotherapy (Reck et al. 2016). Whereas the median progression-free survival was 10.3 months in patients who received pembrolizumab, it was 6.0 months in those who received chemotherapy (HR for disease progression or death 0.50). Patients who received pembrolizumab also had a higher response rate (44.8%) than those who received chemotherapy (27.8%). The duration of response was not reached in those treated with pembrolizumab, and there were fewer treatment-related adverse events. In short, pembrolizumab improves responses rates, duration of response, and survival compared to chemotherapy in patients with 50% or great PD-L1 tumor cell expression. In contrast, a different clinical trial compared nivolumab to platinum-based chemotherapy in patients with 1% or greater tumor cell expression of PD-L1 as detected by the 28–8 clone; however, the primary endpoint was progression-free survival amongst patients with 5% or greater PD-L1 expression. The median progression-free survival was 4.2 months in the group of patients that received nivolumab and 5.9 months in the group that received chemotherapy (HR for disease progression or death 1.15). In an exploratory analysis, it was shown that patients with a high mutation burden (defined as 243 or more mutations) had an improved mprogression-free survival when treated with nivolumab (9.7 months) compared to those treated with chemotherapy (5.8 months; HR 0.62). Conversely, patients with a low (defined as 0–99 mutations) or medium (defined as 100–242 mutations) mutation burden had an inferior mprogression-free survival when treated with nivolumab (4.1 months) compared to those treated with chemotherapy (6.9 months; HR 1.82). It is worth emphasizing that the tumor mutation burden analysis has not been approved for use as a diagnostic test and is exploratory; however, it has some encouraging potential to select patients and will be discussed in more detail below. It is challenging to state with certainty why the frontline trial of pembrolizumab was successful but that of nivolumab was not, as these two agents target the same molecule. In the end, the major differences between the trials other than the agents themselves were the PD-L1 clones used for immunohistochemistry, and the cut-off applied to determine a positive case. As frontline approvals currently stand, pembrolizumab may be used for the treatment of patients with 50% or greater tumor cell PD-L1 expression.

Pembrolizumab has also received accelerated approval by the FDA for treatment of NSCLC-adenocarcinomas in combination with carboplatin and pemetrexed (Langer et al. 2016). In the clinical trial that led to this approval, patients who were stratified by PD-L1 tumor cell expression (< 1% compared to ≥ 1%) were randomized to chemotherapy alone, or chemotherapy with pembrolizumab. Those who received chemotherapy alone could receive maintenance pemetrexed indefinitely, and those who received the combination of chemotherapy with pembrolizumab could receive maintenance pemetrexed indefinitely and pembrolizumab for up 24 months. Only 123 patients participated in this trial; however, the response rate was significantly higher for the group receiving pembrolizumab with chemotherapy (55%) than chemotherapy alone (29%), albeit with more toxicity (39% vs. 26%, respectively). Response rates of patients treated with pembrolizumab and chemotherapy varied by PD-L1 tumor cell expression, such that the response rate of those with < 1% expression was 57%, those with ≥ 1% expression was 54%, those with 1–49% expression was 26%, and those with ≥ 50% expression was 80%. Accordingly, the expression of PD-L1 seems to enrich for responses when a higher cut-off is used.

Atezolizumab

Atezolizumab (also known as MPDL3280A) is a humanized, IgG1 monoclonal antibody that targets PD-L1. The phase 2 POPLAR trial randomly assigned 287 patients with squamous (34%) and non-squamous (66%) NSCLC who had progressed on prior platinum-based therapy to receive either atezolizumab 1,200 mg every 3 weeks or docetaxel (Fehrenbacher et al. 2016). Whereas nivolumab and pembrolizumab target PD-1, which is more commonly detected on T cells than tumor cells, atezolizumab targets PD-L1. While the complementary and companion diagnostics tests of PD-L1 for nivolumab and pembrolizumab have focused on PD-L1 expression by cancer cells, the POPLAR study with atezolizumab investigated PD-L1 expression on tumor cells (TC) and tumor-infiltrating immune cells (IC). Accordingly, subjects who participated in POPLAR had PD-L1 expression scored semi-quantitatively as IC 0, 1, 2, or 3 and TC 0, 1, 2, or 3. Overall survival was significantly better for subjects treated with atezolizumab (12.6 months, 95% CI 9.7–16.4) than those treated with docetaxel (9.7 months, 95% CI 8.6–12). Even though the objective response rates were the same for the two groups (15%), the responses were more durable with atezolizumab, (14.4 months, 95% CI 11.6–nonestimable) than with docetaxel (7.2 months, 95% CI 5.6–12.5). POPLAR included 97 patients with squamous NSCLC, and in this group overall survival was 10.1 months in the atezolizumab group and 8.6 months in the docetaxel group (HR 0.80; 0.49–1.30). In the 190 patients with non-squamous NSCLC, overall survival was 15.5 months in the atezolizumab group and 10.9 months in the docetaxel group (HR 0.69; 95% CI 0.47–1.01). There was a predictive benefit for atezolizumab with increasing PD-L1 expression by TC, IC, or both. Patients in the TC2/3 or IC2/3 subgroups treated with atezolizumab had an improved overall survival (15.1 months, 95% CI 8.4–non-estimable) compared with patients receiving docetaxel (7.4 months, 95% CI 6–12.5). In contrast, patients with PD-L1 levels less than 1% (TC0 and IC0 groups) did not appear to benefit from atezolizumab and had the same survival as subjects treated with docetaxel (9.7 months). This study also looked into the T-cell effector-associated and interferon-γ-associated gene expression signatures, and they both were found to correlate with PD-L1 expression by IC but not by TC. Atezolizumab improved overall survival in patients with tumors with high expression T-cell-effector associated and interferon-γ associated genes and high expression of other genes associated with the PD-L1: PD-1 pathway (PD-L1 receptors *PD-1* and *B7.1*, and the alternative ligand, *PD-L2*). Grade 3–5 adverse events were less common in patients treated with atezolizumab (40%) compared with patients treated with docetaxel (53%). The most common treatment-related AEs of any grade reported for atezolizumab were fatigue (20.4%), decreased appetite (17.6%), and nausea (12%). Pneumonitis of any grade was reported in 3% of patients. POPLAR was the first study to show the promising safety and the efficacy of PD-L1 blockade in second- or third-line treatment of NSCLC and demonstrated the predictive use of PD-L1 expression by TC and IC.

Subsequent to the POPLAR trial, the OAK trial randomized patients who had received 1–2 prior treatments to atezolizumab or docetaxel (Rittmeyer et al. 2017). The primary endpoint was overall survival in the intention-to-treat population and in the PD-L1 expression groups (TC 1/2/3 or IC 1/2/3, $\geq$ 1% PD-L1 expression on tumor cells or tumor-infiltrating immune cells). The primary efficacy analysis was performed on 850 of the 1,225 enrolled patients. Overall survival was significantly better amongst patients who received atezolizumab (median 13.8 months) than docetaxel (median 9.6 months; HR 0.73; 95% CI 0.62–0.87, p=0.0003). Although overall survival in the TC 1/2/3 or IC 1/2/3 population was even better amongst patients who received atezolizumab (median 15.7 months) than docetaxel (median 10.3 months; HR 0.74; 95% CI 0.58–0.93, p=0.0102), overall survival was also better in the PD-L1 undetectable group for patients treated with atezolizumab (median 12.6 months) than docetaxel (median 8.9 months; HR 0.75; 95% CI 0.59–0.96). This survival benefit was seen regardless of histology. Less toxicity was observed with atezolizumab than docetaxel. In previously treated NSCLC, atezolizumab improves survival with a better safety profile compared to docetaxel.

Small Cell Lung Cancer

Most of the recent discoveries and advances in lung cancer treatment have focused on NSCLC and the approach to SCLC has not changed significantly for decades. The encouraging responses to immunotherapy seen in NSCLC and other malignancies have prompted the study of this treatment for SCLC. A phase 1/2 clinical trial for SCLC tested nivolumab or nivolumab and ipilimumab in patients with progression after a platinum-containing regimen. Patients who received nivolumab alone were treated at 3 mg/kg every 2 weeks, whereas those who received the combination of nivolumab and ipilimumab received 1 mg/kg plus 1 mg/kg or 1 mg/kg plus 3 mg/kg or 3 mg/kg plus 1 mg/kg, respectively, every 3 weeks, followed by nivolumab 3 mg/kg every 2 weeks. The trial was ongoing at the time of publication, but the data for 216 patients were reported with response rates varying from 10% for nivolumab alone, to 33% (1/3) in patients receiving 1 mg/kg of nivolumab with 1 mg/kg of ipilimumab, to 23% (14/61) of patients receiving 1 mg/kg of nivolumab and 3 mg/kg of ipilimumab (Antonia et al. 2016). Responses were observed regardless of PD-L1 expression. Given the response rates seen with the commonly used second-line agent topotecan (Von Pawel et al. 2014), these results strongly encourage the use of combined CTLA-4 and PD-1 inhibition in SCLC. Although this combination has not yet been approved by the FDA, its use is recommended by the National Comprehensive Cancer Network as of March 2017. Other drugs such as pembrolizumab are also being tested in SCLC.

Endpoints in Immunotherapy Trials for Non-Small-Cell Lung Cancer

Soon after the CTLA-4 inhibitor ipilimumab was introduced for the treatment of melanoma it was recognized that there are distinct response patterns associated with favorable survival including responses after a radiographic increase in tumor size and appearance of new lesions (pseudoprogression). These observations led to the introduction of the Immune-Related Response Criteria (irRC) instead of Response Evaluation Criteria in Solid Tumors, version 1.1 (RECIST v1.1) for the assessment of the efficacy of immunotherapy in melanoma (Wolchok et al. 2009). Recently a study focusing on melanoma patients in the KEYNOTE-001 study treated with pembrolizumab compared the responses measured by irRC and RECIST v1.1. It was found that there was a discrepancy in the 2-year overall survival rates depending on the criteria used to determine progressive disease (37.5% in patients with progressive disease per RECIST v1.1 but non-progressive disease per irRC, compared with 17.3% in patients with progressive disease per both criteria). Thus, identification of progression per RECIST v1.1 can lead to premature discontinuation of immunotherapy and may deprive patients of additional benefit (Hodi et al. 2016). It is estimated that immune-related radiologic responses—including pseudoprogression—have an overall incidence of 4% in the first immune checkpoint trials, but this calculation can be an underestimation because irRc were not evaluated across all patients (Chiou and Burotto 2015). The existing data are even more scant for NSCLC, and there is an unquantified report of immune-related radiologic responses in NSCLC patients in a study with multiple malignancies (Topalian et al. 2012). Overall it seems that pseudoprogression is not as common in NSCLC as it is in melanoma, but still clinicians should consider it as a possibility until more extensive reporting of the immune-related responses in the current clinical trial will clarify this phenomenon. Clinically, it can be challenging to separate out patients with pseudoprogression from true progression. The decision to continue therapy will depend on other factors such as tolerance of therapy and goals of care.

The novel immunotherapeutic strategies used in the treatment of NSCLC have a mechanism of action that is distinct from the classic cytotoxic chemotherapies. Immunotherapy typically does not have any immediate or direct cytotoxic effects but indirectly acts against tumors by mobilizing the immune system. Nevertheless, the phase 2 and 3 clinical trials of immunotherapy have used the same efficacy endpoints (overall survival, progression-free survival, time to progression, overall response) that have been well established in the evaluation of classic cytotoxic agents. In CheckMate 057 the progression-free survival benefit, in an intention-to-treat analysis, was initially no different or slightly better for docetaxel than nivolumab. It was only after the 8-month mark that nivolumab appeared to be superior, primarily due to the duration of response of the patients who benefited from this agent. The progression-free and overall survival benefits clearly favored nivolumab for patients with detectable PD-L1 expression.

For cytotoxic agents, the progression-free survival usually correlates with overall survival (Suzuki et al. 2015), but this observation does not always hold, possibly due to crossover and the advent of targeted therapies (Hotta et al. 2013; Blumenthal et al. 2015). Since the first studies of immunotherapy, it was noted that the lack of a benefit for progression-free survival does not exclude a significant overall survival benefit—as seen in the CheckMate, KEYNOTE, and POPLAR clinical trials. Thus, for immunotherapy trials, the use of immune-related progression-free survival and overall survival may be more appropriate when judging the efficacy of a new agent (Johnson et al. 2015).

The introduction of immunotherapeutic agents in clinical trials motivates us to re-evaluate our current metrics for a successful trial. Another unique characteristic of the immunotherapy trials is that, usually, the treatment groups do not begin to separate until many months after randomization, while in trials with cytotoxic agents the treatment arms usually would separate soon after randomization. The existing methods that are used for progression-free survival and overall survival are based on the Kaplan Meier method, which assumes that the hazards for the groups under comparison are constant over time. However, in immunotherapy trials, the survival benefit is mainly seen at the tail of the curves many months after randomization. Accordingly, new statistical tools have been proposed (e.g., using the weighted log-rank test, performing additional sensitivity analyses, or estimating survival rates at later rather than usual time points). These statistical tools account for long survivors and late responses (Dranitsaris et al. 2015).

PD-L1 Assessment and Companion Assays

Each of the three FDA-approved PD-1 or PD-L1 inhibitors for NSCLC has a different diagnostic test associated with it for the detection of PD-L1 expression (Table 4.1). Each of the clones used to detect PD-L1 has its own staining characteristics, and its own cut-off for positivity. Given the use of variable cut-offs for PD-L1 expression, and different clones for PD-L1 detection, there is significant confusion over the ideal strategy to test for PD-L1 expression in the clinic (Mansfield and Dong 2016). This confusion is confounded by variable agreement between the assays, intratumoral and intertumoral agreement.

Assay Agreement

Many investigators have assessed how well assays for PD-L1 agree with one another. In one effort, the clones associated with the FDA-approved PD-1 or PD-L1 inhibitors and SP263 were compared to one another amongst 40 NSCLC specimens (Hirsch et al. 2017). The 22C3, 29–8, and SP263 clones similarly detected tumor cell expression; however, SP-142 typically underscored the other clones. Conversely, the SP-142 clone typically detected immune cell PD-L1 expression at higher levels than the other clones. This discrepancy might be because the 28–8, 22C3, and SP142 clones detect extracellular epitopes of PD-L1, and SP142 detects an intracellular epitope. When the respective cut-offs of PD-L1 expression for each clone were applied, 14/38 specimens (37%) were discrepantly categorized. These same four clones were also tested amongst multiple academic institutions using 90 archival NSCLC specimens. In this study, the SP142 clone detected lower PD-L1 expression in tumor cells and immune cells than the other clones. There was better agreement amongst the clones for tumor cell expression than immune cell expression of PD-L1. Agreement between pathologists was very good overall (Rimm et al. 2017). In another study, the 22C3, 28–8, and SP263 clones were tested in 500 archival NSCLC specimens and 90% or better agreement was observed at multiple expression cut-offs (Ratcliffe et al. 2017). These studies suggest that the agreement between most assays for PD-L1 is good overall, but some clones have different patterns of detection, and application of cut-offs can affect agreement.

Table 4.1 US Food and Drug Administration-approved agents and their assays

Agent	Line	Clone	Platform	Cutoff
Nivolumab	≥ 2	28–8	Autostainer Link 48	$\geq 1\%$ tumor cell
Pembrolizumab	≥ 1	22C3	Autostainer Link 48	$\geq 50\%$ tumor cells
Atezolizumab	≥ 2	SP142	BenchMark ULTRA	TC 1/2/3, IC 1/2/3

Heterogeneity

The heterogeneity of PD-L1 expression in lung cancer and other malignancies may affect its applicability as a predictive biomarker. One team of investigators compared PD-L1 expression using the SP142 clone between completely resected lung cancers and matched biopsy specimens. The overall discordance rate was 48% with a kappa value (κ) of 0.218. Agreement of PD-L1 expression improved between matched pairs when many core biopsies were obtained (Ilie et al. 2016). These results suggest that there is a significant degree of intratumoral heterogeneity in PD-L1 expression, and a biopsy without detectable PD-L1 expression does not exclude the possibility of PD-L1 expression elsewhere.

Since most patients who receive immunotherapy for lung cancer have metastatic disease, we have been interested in the heterogeneity of PD-L1 expression between paired lesions. Accordingly, we assessed the agreement of PD-L1 expression between fully resected multifocal lung cancer specimens from 32 patients. Overall, we observed agreement of PD-L1 expression by the tumor cells in paired lesions of 20 patients and disagreement of PD-L1 expression by the tumor cells in paired lesions of 12 patients (κ = 0.01). The expression of PD-L1 is heterogeneous among paired independent lung cancers, but there are high levels of agreement in intrapulmonary metastasis. We used mate-pair sequencing to determine whether these paired multifocal lung cancers were related or not (Mansfield et al. 2016b), and found that 23 patients had independent primary lung cancers and that nine patients had related cancers (intrapulmonary metastases). Amongst the paired lesions from patients with related lung cancers, there was agreement of PD-L1 expression by the tumor cells in eight patients and disagreement in one patient (κ = 0.73). We concluded that the expression of PD-L1 is heterogeneous among paired independent lung cancers, but agreement improves amongst cases of intrapulmonary metastasis (Mansfield et al. 2016b).

In a subsequent project, we assessed the agreement of PD-L1 expression between fully resected primary lung cancers and brain metastases from 73 patients. We observed disagreement of tumor cell PD-L1 expression in 10 cases (14%, κ = 0.71), and disagreement of tumor-infiltrating lymphocyte PD-L1 expression in 19 cases (26%, κ = 0.38) (Fig. 4.1) (Mansfield et al. 2016a). We additionally assessed tumor infiltrating lymphocytes and scored the paired lesions by an immunologic classification schema that others have proposed (Table 4.2) (Teng et al. 2015). Brain metastases commonly lost PD-L1 expression or tumor-infiltrating lymphocytes that were detected in the paired resected specimens, resulting in frequent changes in the immunologic categorizations between primary and metastatic lesions. In summary, the intratumoral and intertumoral heterogeneity of PD-L1 expression may limit the use of PD-L1 expression as a predictive biomarker. Although high PD-L1 expression may enrich for responses to immunotherapy, the lack of PD-L1 expression may not preclude benefit from immunotherapy. Additional work is needed to identify more robust predictors of benefit.

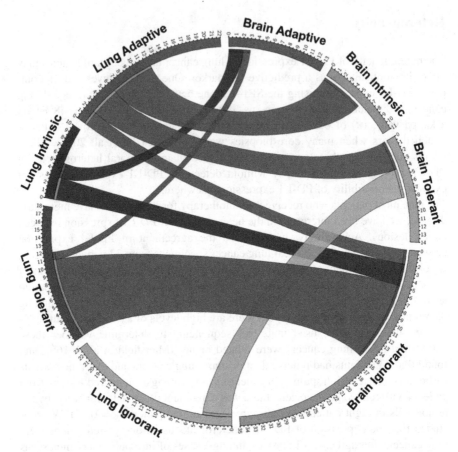

Fig. 4.1 Circos diagram of tumor microenvironment categorizations between paired lesions. The tumor microenvironments of the paired lesions in our series were classified according to Table 4.2 based on tumor-cell expression of PD-L1 and tumor-infiltrating lymphocytes. The circular segments are labeled with these classifications, and the numbers of lesions within each classification are shown with tick marks around the segments. Cases with discordant classifications between the paired primary lung cancers and brain metastases are connected by colored ribbons to demonstrate the dynamics of the discrepant tumor microenvironment classifications between pairs. Concordant cases are not connected by ribbons. Overall, many of the brain metastases lost PD-L1 expression or tumor lymphocyte infiltration that was present in the primary lung cancer specimens (Figure used with permission by Oxford University Press and was previously published elsewhere (Mansfield et al. 2016a))

Table 4.2 Immunologic classification of tumors

	PD-L1+	PD-L1−
TIL+	Adaptive immune resistance	Tolerance (other suppressors)
TIL−	Intrinsic induction	Immunologic ignorance

The immunologic classification is summarized above based on the presence of tumor-cell expression of PD-L1 and tumor-infiltrating lymphocytes (TIL) as proposed by others (Teng et al. 2015).

Other Biomarkers and Future Developments

As novel biomarkers are investigated and developed, it is important to consider where they fit into the steps required for an anti-tumor T-cell response. In this regard, others have proposed analyzing tumors with a cancer immunogram (Blank et al. 2016). This immunogram considers many factors that are required for an effective T-cell response including: tumor foreignness or its mutational load, overall lymphocyte count, presence of intratumoral T cells, absence of immune checkpoint expression, absence of soluble inhibitors, absence of inhibitory tumor metabolism, and tumor sensitivity such as MHC expression. One could imagine that a cancer with a high mutation burden, that presents neoantigens on HLA molecules, that does not express soluble T-cell inhibitors but does express an immune checkpoint, may be responsive to immune checkpoint inhibition. This immunogram also suggests that many components of the immune system and tumor may need to be measured to most accurately predict who will benefit from immunotherapy. In this regard, one group from Japan has started to classify lung cancers with a variation of this immunogram in order to personalize immunotherapy recommendations for patients (Karasaki et al. 2017). This group observed three common immunogram patterns, which suggests that more than one immunologic approach may be necessary moving forward.

Another group has looked at the significance of tumor mutation burden. Their results have suggested that high somatic, non-synonymous mutation burdens are associated with clinical benefit with the PD-1 inhibitor pembrolizumab (Rizvi et al. 2015a). Subsequent work with other investigators demonstrated that clonal neoantigens elicit T-cell immunoreactivity (Mcgranahan et al. 2016). As mentioned above, a retrospective analysis suggested that a high tumor mutation burden is associated with benefit with frontline treatment with the PD-1 inhibitor nivolumab (Carbone et al. 2017), even though 5% or greater PD-L1 expression was not predictive of benefit. When placed in the context of the cancer immunogram mentioned above, a high tumor mutation burden suggests that there are neoantigens that may elicit an anti-tumor T-cell response; however, tumor mutation burden alone ignores the rest of the immunologic milieu that might be needed to select immunotherapy or others as novel therapeutic options become available.

Conclusion

Immunotherapy is rapidly moving forward in lung cancer. Three immunotherapies that target PD-1 or PD-L1 are already approved by the FDA for metastatic NSCLC, and others are in development. These agents are being tested in earlier stages of disease prior to surgery, and in combination with or following chemoradiation. Novel blood-based and tissue biomarkers are being developed and validated. On the preclinical side, better models are being developed that will allow further interrogation of immunologic interplay with lung cancer. Although significant strides have been made so far, many more are to come with patient selection, treatment individualization, and monitoring.

References

Antonia, S. J., Lopez-Martin, J. A., Bendell, J., Ott, P. A., Taylor, M., Eder, J. P., Jager, D., Pietanza, M. C., Le, D. T., De Braud, F., Morse, M. A., Ascierto, P. A., Horn, L., Amin, A., Pillai, R. N., Evans, J., Chau, I., Bono, P., Atmaca, A., Sharma, P., Harbison, C. T., Lin, C. S., Christensen, O., & Calvo, E. (2016). Nivolumab alone and nivolumab plus ipilimumab in recurrent small-cell lung cancer (CheckMate 032): A multicentre, open-label, phase 1/2 trial. *Lancet Oncol, 17*, 883–895.

Blank, C. U., Haanen, J. B., Ribas, A., & Schumacher, T. N. (2016). CANCER IMMUNOLOGY. The "cancer immunogram". *Science, 352*, 658–660.

Blumenthal, G. M., Karuri, S. W., Zhang, H., Zhang, L., Khozin, S., Kazandjian, D., Tang, S., Sridhara, R., Keegan, P., & Pazdur, R. (2015). Overall response rate, progression-free survival, and overall survival with targeted and standard therapies in advanced non-small-cell lung cancer: US Food and Drug Administration trial-level and patient-level analyses. *J Clin Oncol, 33*, 1008–1014.

Boland, J. M., Kwon, E. D., Harrington, S. M., Wampfler, J. A., Tang, H., Yang, P., & Aubry, M. C. (2013). Tumor B7-H1 and B7-H3 expression in squamous cell carcinoma of the lung. *Clinical Lung Cancer, 14*, 157–163.

Borghaei, H., Paz-Ares, L., Horn, L., Spigel, D. R., Steins, M., Ready, N. E., Chow, L. Q., Vokes, E. E., Felip, E., Holgado, E., Barlesi, F., Kohlhäufl, M., Arrieta, O., Burgio, M. A., Fayette, J., Lena, H., Poddubskaya, E., Gerber, D. E., Gettinger, S. N., Rudin, C. M., Rizvi, N., Crinò, L., Blumenschein, G. R. J., Antonia, S. J., Dorange, C., Harbison, C. T., Graf Finckenstein, F., & Brahmer, J. R. (2015). Nivolumab versus docetaxel in advanced nonsquamous non-small-cell lung cancer. *New England Journal of Medicine, 373*, 1627–1639.

Brahmer, J., Reckamp, K. L., Baas, P., Crinò, L., Eberhardt, W. E. E., Poddubskaya, E., Antonia, S., Pluzanski, A., Vokes, E. E., Holgado, E., Waterhouse, D., Ready, N., Gainor, J., Arén Frontera, O., Havel, L., Steins, M., Garassino, M. C., Aerts, J. G., Domine, M., Paz-Ares, L., Reck, M., Baudelet, C., Harbison, C. T., Lestini, B., & Spigel, D. R. (2015). Nivolumab versus docetaxel in advanced squamous-cell non-small-cell lung cancer. *New England Journal of Medicine, 373*, 123–135.

Carbone, D. P., Reck, M., Paz-Ares, L., Creelan, B., Horn, L., Steins, M., Felip, E., Van Den Heuvel, M. M., Ciuleanu, T. E., Badin, F., Ready, N., Hiltermann, T. J. N., Nair, S., Juergens, R., Peters, S., Minenza, E., Wrangle, J. M., Rodriguez-Abreu, D., Borghaei, H., Blumenschein, G. R., Jr., Villaruz, L. C., Havel, L., Krejci, J., Corral Jaime, J., Chang, H., Geese, W. J., Bhagavatheeswaran, P., Chen, A. C., Socinski, M. A., & Checkmate, I. (2017). First-line nivolumab in stage IV or recurrent non-small-cell lung cancer. *N Engl J Med, 376*, 2415–2426.

Chiou, V. L., & Burotto, M. (2015). Pseudoprogression and immune-related response in solid tumors. *J Clin Oncol, 33*, 3541–3543.

Dong, H., Zhu, G., Tamada, K., & Chen, L. (1999). B7-H1, a third member of the B7 family, co-stimulates T-cell proliferation and interleukin-10 secretion. *Nat Med, 5*, 1365–1369.

Dong, H., Strome, S. E., Salomao, D. R., Tamura, H., Hirano, F., Flies, D. B., Roche, P. C., Lu, J., Zhu, G., Tamada, K., Lennon, V. A., Celis, E., & Chen, L. (2002). Tumor-associated B7-H1 promotes T-cell apoptosis: A potential mechanism of immune evasion. *Nat Med, 8*, 793–800.

Dranitsaris, G., Cohen, R. B., Acton, G., Keltner, L., Price, M., Amir, E., Podack, E. R., & Schreiber, T. H. (2015). Statistical considerations in clinical trial design of immunotherapeutic cancer agents. *Journal of Immunotherapy, 38*, 259–266.

Ettinger, D. S., Wood, D. E., Aisner, D. L., Akerley, W., Bauman, J., Chirieac, L. R., D'amico, T. A., Decamp, M. M., Dilling, T. J., Dobelbower, M., Doebele, R. C., Govindan, R., Gubens, M. A., Hennon, M., Horn, L., Komaki, R., Lackner, R. P., Lanuti, M., Leal, T. A., Leisch, L. J., Lilenbaum, R., Lin, J., Loo, B. W., Martins, R., Otterson, G. A., Reckamp, K., Riely, G. J., Schild, S. E., Shapiro, T. A., Stevenson, J., Swanson, S. J., Tauer, K., Yang, S. C., Gregory, K., & Hughes, M. (2017). Non-small cell lung cancer, version 5.2017, NCCN clinical practice guidelines in oncology. *Journal of the National Comprehensive Cancer Network : JNCCN, 15*, 504–535.

Fehrenbacher, L., Spira, A., Ballinger, M., Kowanetz, M., Vansteenkiste, J., Mazieres, J., Park, K., Smith, D., Artal-Cortes, A., Lewanski, C., Braiteh, F., Waterkamp, D., He, P., Zou, W., Chen, D. S., Yi, J., Sandler, A., Rittmeyer, A., & Group, P. S. (2016). Atezolizumab versus docetaxel for patients with previously treated non-small-cell lung cancer (POPLAR): a multicentre, open-label, phase 2 randomised controlled trial. *Lancet, 387*, 1837–1846.

Ferlay, J., Soerjomataram, I., Dikshit, R., Eser, S., Mathers, C., Rebelo, M., Parkin, D. M., Forman, D., & Bray, F. (2015). Cancer incidence and mortality worldwide: sources, methods and major patterns in GLOBOCAN 2012. *Int J Cancer, 136*, E359–E386.

Garon, E. B., Rizvi, N. A., Hui, R., Leighl, N., Balmanoukian, A. S., Eder, J. P., Patnaik, A., Aggarwal, C., Gubens, M., Horn, L., Carcereny, E., Ahn, M.-J., Felip, E., Lee, J.-S., Hellmann, M. D., Hamid, O., Goldman, J. W., Soria, J.-C., Dolled-Filhart, M., Rutledge, R. Z., Zhang, J., Lunceford, J. K., Rangwala, R., Lubiniecki, G. M., Roach, C., Emancipator, K., & Gandhi, L. (2015). Pembrolizumab for the treatment of non-small-cell lung cancer. *New England Journal of Medicine, 372*, 2018–2028.

Gettinger, S. N., Horn, L., Gandhi, L., Spigel, D. R., Antonia, S. J., Rizvi, N. A., Powderly, J. D., Heist, R. S., Carvajal, R. D., Jackman, D. M., Sequist, L. V., Smith, D. C., Leming, P., Carbone, D. P., Pinder-Schenck, M. C., Topalian, S. L., Hodi, F. S., Sosman, J. A., Sznol, M., Mcdermott, D. F., Pardoll, D. M., Sankar, V., Ahlers, C. M., Salvati, M., Wigginton, J. M., Hellmann, M. D., Kollia, G. D., Gupta, A. K., & Brahmer, J. R. (2015). Overall survival and long-term safety of nivolumab (Anti–Programmed Death 1 Antibody, BMS-936558, ONO-4538) in patients with previously treated advanced non–small-cell lung cancer. *Journal of Clinical Oncology, 33*, 2004–2012.

Herbst, R. S., Baas, P., Kim, D. W., Felip, E., Perez-Gracia, J. L., Han, J. Y., Molina, J., Kim, J. H., Arvis, C. D., Ahn, M. J., Majem, M., Fidler, M. J., De Castro, G., Jr., Garrido, M., Lubiniecki, G. M., Shentu, Y., Im, E., Dolled-Filhart, M., & Garon, E. B. (2016). Pembrolizumab versus docetaxel for previously treated, PD-L1-positive, advanced non-small-cell lung cancer (KEYNOTE-010): A randomised controlled trial. *Lancet, 387*, 1540–1550.

Hirsch, F. R., Mcelhinny, A., Stanforth, D., Ranger-Moore, J., Jansson, M., Kulangara, K., Richardson, W., Towne, P., Hanks, D., Vennapusa, B., Mistry, A., Kalamegham, R., Averbuch, S., Novotny, J., Rubin, E., Emancipator, K., Mccaffery, I., Williams, J. A., Walker, J., Longshore, J., Tsao, M. S., & Kerr, K. M. (2017). PD-L1 immunohistochemistry assays for lung cancer: Results from phase 1 of the Blueprint PD-L1 IHC Assay Comparison Project. *Journal of Thoracic Oncology, 12*, 208–222.

Hodi, F. S., Hwu, W. J., Kefford, R., Weber, J. S., Daud, A., Hamid, O., Patnaik, A., Ribas, A., Robert, C., Gangadhar, T. C., Joshua, A. M., Hersey, P., Dronca, R., Joseph, R., Hille, D., Xue, D., Li, X. N., Kang, S. P., Ebbinghaus, S., Perrone, A., & Wolchok, J. D. (2016). Evaluation of immune-related response criteria and RECIST v1.1 in patients with advanced melanoma treated with pembrolizumab. *J Clin Oncol, 34*, 1510–1517.

Hotta, K., Suzuki, E., Di Maio, M., Chiodini, P., Fujiwara, Y., Takigawa, N., Ichihara, E., Reck, M., Manegold, C., Pilz, L., Hisamoto-Sato, A., Tabata, M., Tanimoto, M., Shepherd, F. A., & Kiura, K. (2013). Progression-free survival and overall survival in phase III trials of molecular-targeted agents in advanced non-small-cell lung cancer. *Lung Cancer, 79*, 20–26.

Ilie, M., Long-Mira, E., Bence, C., Butori, C., Lassalle, S., Bouhlel, L., Fazzalari, L., Zahaf, K., Lalvée, S., Washetine, K., Mouroux, J., Vénissac, N., Poudenx, M., Otto, J., Sabourin, J. C., Marquette, C. H., Hofman, V., & Hofman, P. (2016). Comparative study of the PD-L1 status between surgically resected specimens and matched biopsies of NSCLC patients reveal major discordances: A potential issue for anti-PD-L1 therapeutic strategies. *Annals of Oncology, 27,* 147–153.

Johnson, P., Greiner, W., Al-Dakkak, I., & Wagner, S. (2015). Which metrics are appropriate to describe the value of new cancer therapies? *BioMed research international, 2015.*

Karasaki, T., Nagayama, K., Kuwano, H., Nitadori, J. I., Sato, M., Anraku, M., Hosoi, A., Matsushita, H., Morishita, Y., Kashiwabara, K., Takazawa, M., Ohara, O., Kakimi, K., & Nakajima, J. (2017). An immunogram for the cancer-immunity cycle: Towards personalized immunotherapy of lung cancer. *J Thorac Oncol, 12,* 791–803.

Langer, C. J., Gadgeel, S. M., Borghaei, H., Papadimitrakopoulou, V. A., Patnaik, A., Powell, S. F., Gentzler, R. D., Martins, R. G., Stevenson, J. P., Jalal, S. I., Panwalkar, A., Yang, J. C., Gubens, M., Sequist, L. V., Awad, M. M., Fiore, J., Ge, Y., Raftopoulos, H., Gandhi, L., & Investigators, K. (2016). Carboplatin and pemetrexed with or without pembrolizumab for advanced, non-squamous non-small-cell lung cancer: A randomised, phase 2 cohort of the open-label KEYNOTE-021 study. *Lancet Oncol, 17,* 1497–1508.

Leventakos, K., & Mansfield, A. S. (2014). Reflections on immune checkpoint inhibition in non-small cell lung cancer. *Transl Lung Cancer Res, 3,* 411–413.

Leventakos, K., & Mansfield, A. S. (2016). Advances in the treatment of non-small cell lung cancer: Focus on nivolumab, pembrolizumab, and atezolizumab. *BioDrugs, 30,* 397–405.

Mansfield, A. S., & Dong, H. (2016). Implications of programmed cell death 1 Ligand 1 heterogeneity in the selection of patients with non-small cell lung cancer to receive immunotherapy. *Clin Pharmacol Ther, 100,* 220–222.

Mansfield, A. S., Aubry, M. C., Moser, J. C., Harrington, S. M., Dronca, R. S., Park, S. S., & Dong, H. (2016a). Temporal and spatial discordance of programmed cell death-ligand 1 expression and lymphocyte tumor infiltration between paired primary lesions and brain metastases in lung cancer. *Annals Of Oncology, 27,* 1953–1958.

Mansfield, A. S., Murphy, S. J., Peikert, T., Yi, E. S., Vasmatzis, G., Wigle, D. A., & Aubry, M. C. (2016b). Heterogeneity of programmed cell death ligand 1 expression in multifocal lung cancer. *Clin Cancer Res, 22,* 2177–2182.

Mcgranahan, N., Furness, A. J., Rosenthal, R., Ramskov, S., Lyngaa, R., Saini, S. K., Jamal-Hanjani, M., Wilson, G. A., Birkbak, N. J., Hiley, C. T., Watkins, T. B., Shafi, S., Murugaesu, N., Mitter, R., Akarca, A. U., Linares, J., Marafioti, T., Henry, J. Y., Van Allen, E. M., Miao, D., Schilling, B., Schadendorf, D., Garraway, L. A., Makarov, V., Rizvi, N. A., Snyder, A., Hellmann, M. D., Merghoub, T., Wolchok, J. D., Shukla, S. A., Wu, C. J., Peggs, K. S., Chan, T. A., Hadrup, S. R., Quezada, S. A., & Swanton, C. (2016). Clonal neoantigens elicit T cell immunoreactivity and sensitivity to immune checkpoint blockade. *Science, 351,* 1463–1469.

Pardoll, D. M. (2012). The blockade of immune checkpoints in cancer immunotherapy. *Nat Rev Cancer, 12,* 252–264.

Ratcliffe, M. J., Sharpe, A., Midha, A., Barker, C., Scott, M., Scorer, P., Al-Masri, H., Rebelatto, M. C., & Walker, J. (2017). Agreement between programmed cell death ligand-1 diagnostic assays across multiple protein expression cutoffs in non-small cell lung cancer. *Clin Cancer Res, 23,* 3585–3591.

Reck, M., Rodríguez-Abreu, D., Robinson, A. G., Hui, R., Csőszi, T., Fülöp, A., Gottfried, M., Peled, N., Tafreshi, A., Cuffe, S., O'brien, M., Rao, S., Hotta, K., Leiby, M. A., Lubiniecki, G. M., Shentu, Y., Rangwala, R., Brahmer, J. R., & Investigators, K. (2016). Pembrolizumab versus chemotherapy for PD-L1-Positive non-small-cell lung cancer. *The New England Journal of Medicine, 375,* 1823–1833.

Rimm, D. L., Han, G., Taube, J. M., Yi, E. S., Bridge, J. A., Flieder, D. B., Homer, R., West, W. W., Wu, H., Roden, A. C., Fujimoto, J., Yu, H., Anders, R., Kowalewski, A., Rivard, C., Rehman, J., Batenchuk, C., Burns, V., Hirsch, F. R., & Wistuba, I. I. (2017). A prospective, multiinstitutional, pathologist-based assessment of 4 immunohistochemistry assays for PD-L1 expression in non-small cell lung cancer. *JAMA Oncology, 3*(8), 1051–1058.

Rittmeyer, A., Barlesi, F., Waterkamp, D., Park, K., Ciardiello, F., Von Pawel, J., Gadgeel, S. M., Hida, T., Kowalski, D. M., Dols, M. C., Cortinovis, D. L., Leach, J., Polikoff, J., Barrios, C., Kabbinavar, F., Frontera, O. A., De Marinis, F., Turna, H., Lee, J. S., Ballinger, M., Kowanetz, M., He, P., Chen, D. S., Sandler, A., Gandara, D. R., & Group, O. A. K. S. (2017). Atezolizumab versus docetaxel in patients with previously treated non-small-cell lung cancer (OAK): A phase 3, open-label, multicentre randomised controlled trial. *Lancet, 389*, 255–265.

Rizvi, N. A., Hellmann, M. D., Snyder, A., Kvistborg, P., Makarov, V., Havel, J. J., Lee, W., Yuan, J., Wong, P., Ho, T. S., Miller, M. L., Rekhtman, N., Moreira, A. L., Ibrahim, F., Bruggeman, C., Gasmi, B., Zappasodi, R., Maeda, Y., Sander, C., Garon, E. B., Merghoub, T., Wolchok, J. D., Schumacher, T. N., & Chan, T. A. (2015a). Cancer immunology. Mutational landscape determines sensitivity to PD-1 blockade in non-small cell lung cancer. *Science, 348*, 124–128.

Rizvi, N. A., Mazières, J., Planchard, D., Stinchcombe, T. E., Dy, G. K., Antonia, S. J., Horn, L., Lena, H., Minenza, E., Mennecier, B., Otterson, G. A., Campos, L. T., Gandara, D. R., Levy, B. P., Nair, S. G., Zalcman, G., Wolf, J., Souquet, P.-J., Baldini, E., Cappuzzo, F., Chouaid, C., Dowlati, A., Sanborn, R., Lopez-Chavez, A., Grohe, C., Huber, R. M., Harbison, C. T., Baudelet, C., Lestini, B. J., & Ramalingam, S. S. (2015b). Activity and safety of nivolumab, an anti-PD-1 immune checkpoint inhibitor, for patients with advanced, refractory squamous non-small-cell lung cancer (CheckMate 063): A phase 2, single-arm trial. *The Lancet Oncology, 16*, 257–265.

Siegel, R. L., Miller, K. D., & Jemal, A. (2017). Cancer Statistics, 2017. *CA Cancer J Clin, 67*, 7–30.

Suzuki, H., Hirashima, T., Okamoto, N., Yamadori, T., Tamiya, M., Morishita, N., Shiroyama, T., Takeoka, S., Osa, A., Azuma, Y., & Kawase, I. (2015). Relationship between progression-free survival and overall survival in patients with advanced non-small cell lung cancer treated with anticancer agents after first-line treatment failure. *Asia Pac J Clin Oncol, 11*, 121–128.

Teng, M. W., Ngiow, S. F., Ribas, A., & Smyth, M. J. (2015). Classifying cancers based on T-cell infiltration and PD-L1. *Cancer Research, 75*, 2139–2145.

Topalian, S. L., Hodi, F. S., Brahmer, J. R., Gettinger, S. N., Smith, D. C., Mcdermott, D. F., Powderly, J. D., Carvajal, R. D., Sosman, J. A., Atkins, M. B., Leming, P. D., Spigel, D. R., Antonia, S. J., Horn, L., Drake, C. G., Pardoll, D. M., Chen, L., Sharfman, W. H., Anders, R. A., Taube, J. M., Mcmiller, T. L., Xu, H., Korman, A. J., Jure-Kunkel, M., Agrawal, S., Mcdonald, D., Kollia, G. D., Gupta, A., Wigginton, J. M., & Sznol, M. (2012). Safety, activity, and immune correlates of anti-PD-1 antibody in cancer. *N Engl J Med, 366*, 2443–2454.

Velcheti, V., Schalper, K. A., Carvajal, D. E., Anagnostou, V. K., Syrigos, K. N., Sznol, M., Herbst, R. S., Gettinger, S. N., Chen, L., & Rimm, D. L. (2014). Programmed death ligand-1 expression in non-small cell lung cancer. *Lab Invest, 94*, 107–116.

Von Pawel, J., Jotte, R., Spigel, D. R., O'brien, M. E., Socinski, M. A., Mezger, J., Steins, M., Bosquee, L., Bubis, J., Nackaerts, K., Trigo, J. M., Clingan, P., Schutte, W., Lorigan, P., Reck, M., Domine, M., Shepherd, F. A., Li, S., & Renschler, M. F. (2014). Randomized phase III trial of amrubicin versus topotecan as second-line treatment for patients with small-cell lung cancer. *J Clin Oncol, 32*, 4012–4019.

Wolchok, J. D., Hoos, A., O'day, S., Weber, J. S., Hamid, O., Lebbe, C., Maio, M., Binder, M., Bohnsack, O., Nichol, G., Humphrey, R., & Hodi, F. S. (2009). Guidelines for the evaluation of immune therapy activity in solid tumors: Immune-related response criteria. *Clin Cancer Res, 15*, 7412–7420.

Chapter 5
Genitourinary Malignancies

Roxana Dronca and Anagha Bangalore Kumar

Contents

Bladder Cancer

Introduction

Bladder cancer is the most common malignancy involving the urinary system. In the USA, almost 75,000 new cases and 16,000 deaths occur each year due to bladder cancer, making it the fourth most common cancer in men and 11th most common cancer in women (Siegel et al. 2017). Bladder cancer is usually diagnosed in older individuals, usually in the seventh decade of life (Lynch and Cohen 1995), and the

R. Dronca (✉)
Mayo Clinic, Division of Medical Oncology, Rochester, MN, USA

A.B. Kumar
Clinical Pharmacology Fellow, Mayo Clinic, Rochester, MN, USA

© Springer International Publishing AG 2018   79
H. Dong, S.N. Markovic (eds.), *The Basics of Cancer Immunotherapy*,
https://doi.org/10.1007/978-3-319-70622-1_5

incidence increases with age. The disease is extremely rare in children and young adults, and if present, is usually diagnosed as a low-grade, non-invasive, localized tumor (Linn et al. 1998). Smoking and environmental or occupational exposures account for most cases of bladder cancer. Individuals with recurrent or chronic bladder infections and those who have an ongoing source of bladder inflammation (such as neurogenic bladder with or without prolonged indwelling catheters, bladder calculi, Schistosoma infections) also have a higher risk of bladder cancer compared to the general population, especially squamous cell carcinoma. With carcinogen exposure, it is hypothesized that the lining of the entire urinary tract (urothelium) is exposed to substances that are either excreted in the urine or activated from precursors in the urine, which explains the "field effect" seen with urothelial carcinomas of both the urinary bladder and upper urinary tract. Indeed, these tumors tend to be either multifocal at diagnosis or have a high tendency of recurrence over time. As a consequence, many bladder cancer patients experience multiple recurrences over their lifetime, resulting in a relatively large number of bladder cancer survivors currently alive in the USA.

Bladder Cancer Grading and Staging

The treatment and prognosis of bladder cancer depend upon its stage, grade, and the risk that the cancer will recur. Bladder cancer staging is based upon how far the cancer has penetrated into the bladder wall, whether the cancer involves regional (pelvic) lymph nodes, and whether the cancer has spread beyond the bladder to other organs. Tumor grade refers to the microscopic characteristics of the cancer cells; bladder tumors are classified by pathologists as either low or high grade. At diagnosis, about 75% of patients have early-stage, non-muscle-invasive bladder cancer (NMIBC), and only about 25% have more advanced, muscle-invasive disease localized to the bladder or presenting with lymph nodes or distant metastases (Kamat et al. 2016). The risk of recurrence of NMIBC is approximately 50–70% at 5 years and the reported risk of progression to invasive tumors ranges from 10% to 30% (Kamat et al. 2016). The main factors influencing recurrence and progression in superficial (non-invasive) bladder cancer include high grade, high stage, presence of carcinoma in situ, large tumor size, multifocality, and a high number of previous recurrences (Kamat et al. 2016). Invasive bladder cancer is defined as a bladder tumor that has invaded at least the muscularis propria; the main determinant of prognosis for invasive tumors is based on the depth of the tumor invasion, involvement of regional/pelvic lymph nodes, and presence of distant metastases. Patients with nodal metastases but without disseminated disease may be treated with cystectomy or combined-modality approaches, while the presence of distant metastases is considered incurable disease and is generally treated with systemic therapies.

Role of Immunotherapy in the Management of Bladder Cancer

Role of BCG in the Treatment of Non-Muscle-Invasive Bladder Cancer

The initial step in the management of non-muscle-invasive bladder cancer is transurethral resection of all visible tumors with adequate surgical margins using a cystoscopic approach. Further management is based on risk stratification using clinical and pathologic characteristics that classify NMIBC as low risk, intermediate risk, or high risk (Kamat et al. 2016). Because of the high recurrence rate of NMIBC, adjuvant (additional) therapy is usually recommended. The most common and oldest immunotherapy used for bladder cancer is intravesical bacillus Calmette-Guérin (BCG) instillation. BCG is an attenuated live bacterium that causes cow tuberculosis. Although the mechanism of action of BCG is not fully elucidated, animal experiments showed that intravesical BCG was effective against superficial bladder tumors; the first human study with this agent was reportedly conducted in the mid-1970s (Morales et al. 1976). The anti-tumor effects of BCG seem to be the result of direct effects on tumor cells by BCG infection and also activation of the host's immune response (Fuge et al. 2015), which improves the recognition and subsequent destruction of tumor cells through non-specific and specific cell-mediated mechanisms (Alexandroff et al. 1999). It has also been shown that BCG has a predilection for entering bladder cells, and this step seems to be critical for expression of antigen-presenting molecules and the development of a subsequent immune response. Cytokine release, particularly Th1 cytokines (interleukin (IL)-2, tumor necrosis factor, IL-12, and interferon (IFNγ)) along with IL-8 and IL-17, induces anti-tumor activity mediated by not only cytotoxic T lymphocytes, but also natural killer cells, neutrophils, and macrophages (Fuge et al. 2015).Therefore, intravesical BCG, in combination with TURBT, is currently considered to be the most effective treatment for NMIBC and has been shown to delay tumor progression and reduce recurrences (Sylvester et al. 2005). As a result, patients with a high risk of recurrence as well as certain patients with intermediate risk are often advised to start intravesical BCG, usually within 2–6 weeks of the first treatment. This is commonly followed by additional booster treatments (maintenance therapy) once a complete response is obtained. Maintenance therapy improves outcomes when given at full doses for 3 years for patients with high-risk disease, while for some intermediate-risk NMIBC patients 1 year of maintenance treatment was found to be sufficient (Brausi et al. 2014).

Role of Immunotherapy in the Management of Metastatic Bladder Cancer

Until recently, the survival of patients with advanced or metastatic bladder cancer who progressed on, or were not eligible for, conventional platinum-based chemotherapeutic regimens, was extremely limited. In the last few years, multiple clinical trials have been undertaken to evaluate the role of novel immune checkpoint inhibitors in metastatic urothelial carcinoma (mUC), and as a result, several new agents are currently approved by the US Food and Drug Administration (FDA) for this indication.

Atezolizumab is a humanized anti-PDL1 inhibitor that was first reported to be safe and effective in advanced urothelial carcinoma by Powles and colleagues (Powles et al. 2014). This was a phase 1 expansion study, with an adaptive design, that allowed for biomarker-positive enriched cohorts and found that tumors expressing PD-L1-positive tumor-infiltrating immune cells had particularly high response rates. Moreover, the responses were often rapid, with many occurring by the first imaging assessment at 6 weeks, and also durable compared to historically treated chemotherapy patients. The favorable toxicity profile, including a lack of peripheral neuropathy, hearing or renal impairment suggested that this drug may be better tolerated by older patients with bladder cancer compared to chemotherapy. On the basis of these data, the FDA granted atezolizumab breakthrough status for mUC. These results were expanded in the phase 2 IMvigor210 study, which tested treatment with atezolizumab at a dose of 1,200 mg every 3 weeks in two cohorts: the first cohort included cisplatin-ineligible patients with locally advanced or metastatic disease, and cohort 2 consisted of cisplatin-pretreated patients. The results of cohort 2, in which 310 patients with metastatic urothelial cancer were treated with atezolizumab, showed that the objective response rate (ORR) was 15%; in addition, similar to the phase 1 findings, 38 of 45 (84%) responses were ongoing at a median follow-up of 12 months (Rosenberg et al. 2016). In this study, patients' tumor samples were analyzed for PD-L1 expression by the immune cells infiltrating the tumors. The PD-L1 tumor-infiltrating immune-cell (IC) status was defined by the percentage of PD-L1-positive immune cells in the tumor microenvironment as IC0 (< 1% positive cells), IC1 (≥ 1% but < 5% positive cells), and IC2/3 (≥ 5% positive cells). Patients with higher PD-L1 expression had better outcomes; for all evaluable patients, the objective response rate was 15%, with a complete response recorded in 15 (5%) of 310 patients and in the IC2/3 group the objective response rate was 26%, including 11 (11%) patients who achieved a complete response. After a median follow-up of 11.7 months, the median survival for groups IC2/3, IC1 and IC0 were 11.4, 6.7, and 6.4 months, respectively. The most common adverse effect was fatigue, which was seen in 16% of patients. Severe grade 3 and 4 adverse effects were seen in 5% of patients and included abnormal liver function tests, rash, dyspnea, and pneumonitis. Based on these results, the FDA granted atezolizumab accelerated approval for use in patients with locally advanced or metastatic urothelial carcinoma who have disease progression during or following treatment with platinum-based chemotherapy for metastatic disease, or who have disease progression within 1 year of neoadjuvant or adjuvant treatment with platinum-containing chemotherapy. Cohort 1 patients were chemotherapy-naïve patients considered unfit for cisplatin therapy. 119 patients were enrolled under this cohort, 18% had received neo-adjuvant treatment and 10% had radiotherapy. The ORR was 23% and complete responses (CR) were seen in 9% of patients. Median duration of response had not been reached, and 19 of 27 continued to respond at the time of analysis. Median overall survival (OS) for the entire cohort was 15.9 months. Tumor mutation load was associated with response in this study. Immune-mediated all-grade adverse events were reported in 12% of patients and grade 3 and 4 adverse effects occurred in 7%. (Balar et al. 2017) The results of this study subsequently led to the accelerated approval of atezolizumab for frontline treatment of patients with locally advanced or metastatic urothelial carcinoma who are ineligible for cisplatin chemotherapy.

Nivolumab is a fully human monoclonal antibody targeting PD-1. In a phase 1 trial (CheckMate 032), nivolumab was administered at 3 mg/kg every 2 weeks in patients with mUC regardless of PD-L1 status. Of the 86 patients who had enrolled in the study, 78 received at least one dose of the drug; in this cohort, the ORR was 24.4%, median progression-free survival (PFS) 28 months, and survival at 12 months was 51.6%. Grade 3–4 treatment-related adverse events occurred in 17 (22%) of 78 patients (Sharma et al. 2016). A larger single-arm phase 2 study, CheckMate 275, studied nivolumab as a single agent in 270 patients with locally advanced or metastatic urothelial carcinoma who had progressed following platinum-based chemotherapy. Objective responses were seen in 19.6% of patients. Higher levels of PD-L1 expression on tumor cells were associated with higher objective response rates (28.4% with PD-L1 expression > 5%; 23.8% with PD-L1 expression ≥ 1%; and 16.1% with PD-L1 expression < 1%) (Sharma et al. 2017). Based on these data, the FDA granted nivolumab accelerated approval for use in patients with locally advanced or metastatic urothelial carcinoma who have disease progression during or following treatment with platinum-based chemotherapy for metastatic disease, or who have disease progression within 1 year of neoadjuvant or adjuvant treatment with platinum-containing chemotherapy.

Durvalumab is a human anti-PD-L 1 inhibitor that is indicated at the dose of 10 mg/kg intravenously every 2 weeks for the treatment of advanced urothelial carcinoma that has progressed during or after previous platinum-based chemotherapy. Durvalumab was studied in a phase 1/2 trial that included 191 patients (Powles et al. 2017); all but one patient had received prior chemotherapy, which was platinum-based in 95% of cases. Objective responses were seen in 18% (34 patients), including seven complete responses and 27 partial responses. The response rate was higher in tumors with high PD-L1 expression as compared with low or negative PD-L1 expression (28% vs. 5%). Median PFS and OS were 1.5 months and 18.2 months, respectively; the 1-year OS rate was 55%. Grade 3/4 treatment-related adverse events were seen in 7% of patients and there were two immune-mediated adverse events leading to death (autoimmune hepatitis, pneumonitis). Durvalumab achieved FDA approval in May 2017 for locally advanced or metastatic urothelial carcinoma who have progressed during or after treatment with platinum-based chemotherapy or those who progressed within 1 year of neoadjuvant or adjuvant treatment with platinum-containing chemotherapy (Massard et al. 2016).

Avelumab is a humanized anti PD-L1 inhibitor. As part of the phase 1 JAVELIN solid tumor trial (Apolo et al. 2017), 44 patients with mUC were treated with avelumab and followed for a median of 16.5 months. Grade 3–4 treatment-related adverse events occurred in 7% of patients; the confirmed ORR was 18.2%, median PFS was 11.6 weeks, and the median OS was 13.7 months with a 12-month OS rate of 54.3% (Apolo et al. 2017). Avelumab received accelerated FDA approval in May

2017 for locally advanced or metastatic urothelial carcinoma in patients who progressed while on chemotherapy or within 1 year of neoadjuvant or adjuvant treatment with platinum-containing chemotherapy.

Pembrolizumab is a humanized anti PD-1 antibody. The phase 2 KEYNOTE-052 study (O'Donnell et al. 2017) enrolled 374 patients ineligible for cisplatin chemotherapy who received pembrolizumab at a dose of 200 mg every 3 weeks. In this study, the average age of the study population was 74 years, and a third of patients were older than 80 years. The ORR was 29% for the entire cohort, of which 7% were complete responses. Responses were seen across all major subgroups and were durable; the median duration of response had not been reached at the time of analysis. This was a landmark study that led to the approval of pembrolizumab as a frontline agent in cisplatin-ineligible patients. In the phase 3 Keynote-045 trial, 542 patients who had recurred after or progressed on a platinum-containing regimen were randomly assigned to pembrolizumab (200 mg every 3 weeks for 24 months) or investigator's choice chemotherapy (paclitaxel, docetaxel, or vinflunine) (Bellmunt et al. 2017). The response rate was higher with pembrolizumab than with chemotherapy (21.1% vs. 11.0%), and the OS was also significantly increased with pembrolizumab compared with chemotherapy (median 10.3 vs. 7.4 months). Serious treatment-related adverse events were significantly less frequent with pembrolizumab compared to chemotherapy (15.0% vs. 44%). Following these results, pembrolizumab was granted approval for patients who progressed while on chemotherapy or within 1 year of neoadjuvant or adjuvant treatment with platinum-containing chemotherapy.

Mature results from the KEYNOTE-045 trial presented at the European Society for Medical Oncology (ESMO) 2017 Congress confirmed significantly longer survival in patients with advanced urothelial cancer who received pembrolizumab after initial chemotherapy compared to investigator's choice of an alternative chemotherapy regimen (Bellmunt et al. 2017). Some other ongoing studies are NCT02625961, which is analyzing the potential of pembrolizumab in muscle non-invasive bladder cancer relapsing after BCG treatment, NCT02690558, which is studying pembrolizumab in combination with gemcitabine and cisplatin as neoadjuvant therapy, and NCT02500121, which is testing the PD-1 inhibitor pembrolizumab as maintenance therapy after initial chemotherapy in metastatic bladder cancer.

Consensus recommendations: Atezolizumab, durvalumab, avelumab, pembrolizumab, and nivolumab are all FDA approved and recommended for patients with locally advanced or metastatic urothelial carcinoma previously treated with platinum-based chemotherapy or who relapsed within 12 months of perioperative platinum-based chemotherapy. Any of these agents may be chosen based on dosing and convenience. Atezolizumab and pembrolizumab are also recommended as first-line agents in patients ineligible for cisplatin therapy. It is of note that for all approvals granted under the accelerated approval pathway based on response rate and duration of response, continued approval may be contingent on evidence of clinical benefit in further trials (Kamat et al. 2017).

Renal Cell Carcinoma

Introduction

Historically known as hypernephroma or "Grawitz tumor", renal cell cancer was originally believed to arise from ectopic adrenal tissue (Grawitz 1883). It was not until late 1950s when the true renal origin of these tumors was unequivocally established (Foot et al. 1951; Oberling et al. 1960), and the term renal cell carcinoma (RCC) was proposed to more accurately describe these malignancies. Eighty-five to ninety percent of all adult kidney cancers originate in the renal parenchyma, while tumors arising in the renal pelvis account for less than 10% of all cases and are usually of transitional urothelial cell type, and these are managed similarly to bladder cancers (Chow et al. 1999). Most parenchymal tumors are clear-cell renal cell carcinomas (ccRCC). Non-clear-cell histologies constitute 20–25% of RCCs; however, this group is quite heterogeneous, with each individual subtype (i.e., papillary, chromophobe, collecting duct, medullary, translocation carcinoma, etc.) being relatively rare and thus difficult to study in large prospective studies. Sarcomatoid carcinoma is not considered a separate entity, but rather a form of rapidly progressing, poor prognosis RCC, as high-grade sarcomatoid changes may be seen in all subtypes.

Kidney cancer accounts for about 4% of cancer incidence and 2% of cancer mortality in the USA, with approximately 64,000 new cases and almost 14,000 deaths recorded from RCC each year (Siegel et al. 2017). In the USA, the incidence rate of RCC is highest in African Americans, compared to whites and Hispanics, while Asians/Pacific Islanders have the lowest incidence rate (about half of other racial/ethnic groups) (Chow and Devesa 2008). The incidence rates are also higher among men than women, with rates previously reported as twice as high for all racial and ethnic origins (Chow and Devesa 2008), although more recent data suggests that the gap may be narrowing (Jemal et al. 2009). In general, men tend to present with larger, higher grade, and higher stage tumors, and they have a higher incidence of regional and metastatic spread (Aron et al. 2008). RCC is commonly diagnosed in the seventh or eighth decade of life, with less than 5–10% of patients presenting before age 40 years (Gillett et al. 2005; Thompson et al. 2008). Recent studies suggest that younger patients are less likely to have ccRCC (Gillett et al. 2005; Thompson et al. 2008) and are more likely to be symptomatic at presentation and be diagnosed at an earlier stage compared to their older counterparts, despite having tumors of similar size (Verhoest et al. 2007). In the USA, the incidence of RCC has risen consistently over time in all races and sex groups (Chow et al. 1999), which has been in part attributed to increased detection of presymptomatic (incidental) tumors through widespread use of imaging modalities such as ultrasonography, computed tomography, and magnetic resonance imaging performed for the diagnostic work-up of other abdominal disorders (Sanchez-Martin et al. 2008). Indeed, RCC is being increasingly diagnosed at an earlier stage, with marked increases in incidence seen in localized stage tumors, particularly small tumors (< 2 cm) and tumors 2–4 cm in size (Chow and Devesa 2008). The diagnosis at an increasingly early stage and small tumor size may have contributed to consistently decreasing mortality rates in recent years in both males and females (Jemal et al. 2009; Levi et al. 2008). In fact, size at diagnosis appears to be a strong predictor of survival, with smaller sizes leading to improved survival, although US registry data showed that the overall 5-year relative survival rate of patients with RCC has improved over time across all disease stages, suggesting a general improvement in the management of these patients (Chow and Devesa 2008).

Extent of Disease

The Tumor, Nodes, Metastasis (TNM) staging system, which is based upon the extent of the primary tumor and the presence or absence of regional lymph node involvement or distant metastases, is used for staging all histologic variants of renal carcinoma. This staging system correlates with prognosis and provides important information for patient management. Because RCC is nowadays more frequently being diagnosed incidentally as a consequence of increased use of imaging procedures for other reasons, two-thirds of patents have localized disease (i.e., confined to the kidney) at presentation, while the rest are divided equally between patients presenting with regional (i.e., spread to regional lymph nodes) or metastatic disease (Kane et al. 2008).

Role of Immunotherapy in the Management of Renal Cell Carcinoma

RCC is a cancer that has long been considered chemoresistant but highly "immunogenic." This came from the observation in the 1960s that some patients with metastatic RCC (mRCC) experienced a unique phenomenon of spontaneous remission of their metastatic tumors after removal of the primary renal cancer (Everson 1964; Hallahan 1959). Additionally, in the 1980s and 1990s, high-dose IL-2 (HD IL-2) was shown to induce complete responses in about 5–7% of patients, most of them being durable and even potential cures (Fyfe et al. 1995; Fisher et al. 2000). Therefore, harnessing the immune system as an anticancer therapy has long been of interest, especially because of the potential for durable responses that are not seen with cytotoxic or targeted therapy. For mRCC, immunotherapy using cytokines such as IL-2 (Fyfe et al. 1995) or IFN-alfa (IFN-α) (Dekernion et al. 1983) had actually been a primary treatment before the development of targeted therapies in 2005, although the clinical benefit was modest and the use was limited by toxicity and, in the case of HD IL-2, the difficulty of administration in a hospital setting. Since 2005, ten agents have been approved for the treatment of patients with metastatic ccRCC, including six agents that target the tyrosine kinase of vascular endothelial growth factor (VEGF) receptors (sorafenib, sunitinib, pazopanib, axitinib, cabozantinib, and lenvatinib), two agents that target mammalian target of rapamycin (mTOR) pathway (temsirolimus and everolimus), a monoclonal antibody against VEGF (bevacizumab), and one against the immune checkpoint programmed cell death protein-1 (PD-1) (nivolumab). With the abundance of new agents, the role for cytokine-based immunotherapy has become significantly more limited, and the new immunotherapy agents such as immune checkpoint inhibitors are increasingly being used in clinical practice. The main challenge remains the lack of good biomarkers to identify patients most likely to benefit from a particular drug or class of drugs, and the lack of clear evidence from randomized data to guide optimal sequencing among the available agents.

The "Past" Cytokines Interleukin-2 and Interferon-α2b

IL-2 and IFNα2b have been the oldest immunotherapy treatments used for mRCC, although the exact mechanism by which they exert anti-tumor activity is unclear. IL-2 is known to stimulate T-cell proliferation and differentiation, with activity on both effector and regulatory T cells (Smith 1980). High-dose IL-2 (HD IL-2) was approved for the treatment of mRCC in 1992, mainly based on summarized data from 255 patients treated in seven clinical trials (Fyfe et al. 1995). The overall response rate (ORR) was 15% (37/255), of which 17 were complete (CR) and 20 were partial (PR) responses, with 60% of patients with PR exhibiting more than 90% reduction in tumor burden. The median duration of response was 54 months, not reached for CR patients, and 20 months for PR patients. The median OS for all 255 patients was 16 months. Subsequent reports with data from a median of 10 years follow-up showed that the majority (60%) of CR patients remained in complete remission, and four PR patients who underwent surgery of residual disease to achieve CR remained disease-free at more than 65 months (Fisher et al. 2000; Rosenberg et al. 1998). IL-2 is a toxic regimen, with severe side effects possibly affecting multiple organ systems, and requiring administration in a hospital setting and in specialized tertiary centers. Therefore, the probability of durable responses must be balanced against the cost, limited access, and toxicity associated with this treatment, and efforts have been made to identify clinical, histologic, and molecular characteristics that can identify the patient subsets that are most likely to benefit from this approach. The Society for Immunotherapy of Cancer (SITC) has published a consensus statement from a convened task force of experts in RCC (Rini et al. 2016), including criteria for HD IL-2. Criteria that have long been established to be associated with a favorable response include adequate heart and lung function; ECOG (Eastern Cooperative Oncology Group) performance status 0–1, age (physiologic vs. chronologic) less than 70 years; and absence of CNS, bone, or liver metastases (Rini et al. 2016).

IFNα2b has been a mainstay in the treatment of RCC for more than 20 years and has been the control arm for the initial clinical trials that led to the approval of anti-VEGF- and mTOR-targeted therapies in RCC. The activity of monotherapy with IFNα was evaluated in several large trials (Negrier et al. 1998; Flanigan et al. 2001), which used a variety of preparations, doses, and schedules. Overall, the response rate was as high as 15%; the median time to response was about 4 months, and most responses were partial and rarely persisted beyond 1 year. IFN is also a difficult drug to use because of the chronic administration as well as the severity and chronicity of side effects. IFN is currently approved in combination with bevacizumab for treatment of patients with mRCC, based on the results of two phase 3 trials comparing the combination to IFN alone (Escudier et al. 2007; Rini et al. 2008). While in these studies the combination had a better response rate (26–31%) compared to IFN alone (13%), there was no evidence of OS benefit to this approach and most physicians do not routinely use this combination.

Novel Immune Checkpoint Inhibitors

Nivolumab: The results of the landmark phase 3 CheckMate 025 trial led to the FDA approval of nivolumab for patients with metastatic RCC who had received prior anti-angiogenic therapy. This was a large, multicenter trial in which 821 patients with advanced RCC who progressed after at least one anti-angiogenic therapy were randomly assigned to nivolumab (3 mg/kg every 2 weeks) or everolimus (10 mg/day). The median OS was 25.0 months on the nivolumab arm and 19.6 months on the everolimus arm. The confirmed response rates were 25% for the nivolumab arm versus 5% for the everolimus arm, and the OS was significantly increased with nivolumab compared with everolimus (median, 25.0 vs. 19.6 months, respectively). In fact, the trial was stopped early based upon improved OS in a planned interim analysis. With regard to toxicity, fewer patients had grade 3 or 4 toxicity with nivolumab compared with everolimus (19% vs. 37%), and a secondary analysis of 706 patients showed that nivolumab was associated with improvement in quality of life compared to patients treated with everolimus, who had a deterioration in quality of life from their baseline (Cella et al. 2016).

Nivolumab was approved for the treatment of metastatic RCC by the FDA in November 2015 on the basis of this trial. The originally approved dose was 3 mg/kg based upon the dose used in the CheckMate 025 trial; however, the FDA has subsequently modified the approved dosage regimen to 240 mg as a flat dose every 2 weeks, based upon population pharmacokinetics and dose/exposure-response analyses.

Pembrolizumab is being evaluated in two randomized phase 2 trials; in one (NCT02089685), pembrolizumab is being evaluated alone and in combination with pegylated IFNα; another study (NCT02014636) is evaluating pembrolizumab as monotherapy or in combination with pazopanib.

Atezolizumab was evaluated in a phase 1 study in RCC; in this study the rate of partial response among 62 evaluable patients was 15%, and the median duration of response was 17 months. Interestingly, the ORR for patients with Fuhrman grade 4 and/or sarcomatoid histology was 22% (Mcdermott et al. 2016).

Nivolumab plus Ipilimumab

The combination of nivolumab (PD-1 inhibitor) and ipilimumab (CTLA-4 inhibitor) was assessed in the phase 1 CheckMate 016 trial in a first- and second-line setting using different doses of the combination (Hammers et al. 2017). Forty-seven patients were treated with nivolumab 3 mg/kg plus ipilimumab 1 mg/kg (N3I1) or nivolumab 1 mg/kg plus ipilimumab 3 mg/kg (N1I3) every 3 weeks for four doses followed by nivolumab monotherapy 3 mg/kg every 2 weeks until progression or toxicity. At a median follow-up of 22.3 months, the confirmed objective response rate was 40.4% in both arms. The 2-year OS was 67.3% and 69.6% in the N3I1 and N1I3 arms, respectively. The lower dose ipilimumab combination was less toxic; grade 3–4 treatment-related adverse events were reported in 38% and 62% of the patients in the N3I1 and N1I3 arms, respectively.

An international multicenter phase 3 trial (CheckMate 214) in which patients with previously untreated advanced or metastatic RCC were randomly assigned to the N3I1 combination of nivolumab plus ipilimumab or to sunitinib was recently shown to result in a greater ORR and prolonged PFS for immunotherapy compared to sunitinib in intermediate- and poor-risk patients (Escudier et al. 2017). In the combination arm, 550 patients were treated with nivolumab at 3 mg/kg plus ipilimumab at 1 mg/kg every 3 weeks for four doses, followed by nivolumab at 3 mg/kg every 2 weeks and in the targeted therapy arm; 546 patients received sunitinib at 50 mg once daily for 4 weeks and 2 weeks off in 6-week cycles. After approximately 17.5 months of follow-up, the ORR in intermediate/poor-risk patients was 41.6% for the nivolumab/ipilimumab combination compared to 26.5% for sunitinib (p <0.0001) with close to 10% of patients receiving immunotherapy achieving complete response compared to 1.2% of patients on sunitinib. Baseline tumor PD-L1 expression was lower in the cohort of patients with favorable risk (11% of patients on combination had PD-L1 levels $\geq$ 1%) compared to 26% of patients at intermediate or poor risk. The ORR in patients having baseline PD-L1 expression $\geq$ 1% was 58% for combination immunotherapy versus 25% with sunitinib, and median PFS was 22.8 months versus 5.9 months, respectively, HR 0.48 (95% CI 0.28–0.82; p = 0.0003). However, in patients at favorable risk, both the ORR and PFS were higher with sunitinib over the combination; the ORR was 29% with nivolumab/ipilimumab versus 52% with sunitinib (p = 0.0002) and median PFS was 15.3 months versus 25.1 months, respectively, hazard ratio (HR) 2.17 (95% confidence interval (CI) 1.46–3.22; p < 0.0001). These data suggest that the combination of nivolumab plus ipilimumab could be considered as a potential first-line treatment for patients with intermediate/poor-risk metastatic RCC, particularly those patients having tumor PD-L1 expression $\geq$ 1%. However, good-risk patients seem to derive more benefit from front-line targeted therapy.

Combined Antiangiogenic plus Checkpoint Inhibitor Therapy

Atezolizumab plus bevacizumab combination was studied in a phase 2 trial of 305 previously untreated patients with locally advanced or metastatic RCC versus sunitinib, with crossover from the single-agent arms to the combination of atezolizumab plus bevacizumab permitted at time of progression (Atkins et al. 2017). With a median follow-up of 20.7 months, ORRs for atezolizumab plus bevacizumab, atezolizumab alone, and sunitinib were 32%, 25%, and 29%, respectively. For patients with PD-L1 expression ≥ 1% the response rates were 46% for the combination versus 28% for atezolizumab. For patients crossing over to the combination after progression on sunitinib the ORR was 28% versus 24% for those who had progressed after atezolizumab. A phase 3 study of atezolizumab and bevacizumab versus sunitinib in previously untreated metastatic RCC patients is currently underway in the first-line setting (NCT02420821).

Pembrolizumab plus axitinib combination was studied in a phase 1 study with an expansion cohort (Atkins 2016). Objective responses were observed in 37/52 patients (71%); however, 94% of patients in this study had some tumor shrinkage. Toxicity was largely related to axitinib, with grade 3 potentially immune-related adverse effects seen in 20% of patients. This combination is currently being compared with sunitinib in a phase 3 trial, KEYNOTE-426 (NCT02853331).

Avelumab plus axitinib—in a phase 1 study 55 treatment-naïve patients with favorable or intermediate-risk advanced RCC were treated with the combination of avelumab and axitinib (Choueiri et al. 2017). The ORR was 58% and the median progression-free survival was 6.7 months. The combination was well tolerated, with the most common immune-related toxicity being hypothyroidism. This combination is currently being compared with sunitinib in a phase 3 trial (NCT02684006).

Role of PD-L1 Testing in Clinical Practice

Identifying biomarkers of sensitivity is vital to inform clinical decision-making, and to help select patients who are most likely to benefit from PD-1 blockade. Tumor-associated PD-L1 has been proposed as a potential biomarker of response to anti-PD-1 therapy; however, durable responses are also observed in patients with PD-L1 negative tumors, calling into question the clinical utility of PD-L1 expression alone as a predictive biomarker. Currently, the data in mUC do not support using PD-L1 immunohistochemistry to select patients for treatment. However, the FDA has approved complementary assays for evaluating PD-L1 expression when considering treatment with atezolizumab (Ventana PD-L1 SP142) and durvalumab (Ventana PD-L1 SP263) because PD-L1 positivity appears to identify a patient population more likely to respond to anti- PD-L1 therapy in the chemotherapy-refractory setting. However, in both cases durable responses were observed in patients even with low levels of PD-L1 expression, albeit at lower frequencies. Similarly, in metastatic

RCC, expression of the PD-1 ligand 1 (PD-L1) on tumor cells was not associated with OS benefit to nivolumab. Possible explanations for these discordant results are the heterogeneous expression of PD-L1 in tumor tissues, and the fact that tumor PD-L1 expression is dynamic and likely modulated by a variety of factors in the tumor microenvironment, which may explain the inability to capture its expression for predictive purposes with a single time point, random tumor biopsy.

References

Alexandroff, A. B., Jackson, A. M., O'Donnell, M. A., & James, K. (1999). BCG immunotherapy of bladder cancer: 20 years on. *Lancet, 353*, 1689–1694.

Apolo, A. B., Infante, J. R., Balmanoukian, A., Patel, M. R., Wang, D., Kelly, K., Mega, A. E., Britten, C. D., Ravaud, A., Mita, A. C., Safran, H., Stinchcombe, T. E., Srdanov, M., Gelb, A. B., Schlichting, M., Chin, K., & Gulley, J. L. (2017). Avelumab, an anti-programmed death-ligand 1 antibody, in patients with refractory metastatic urothelial carcinoma: results from a multicenter, phase Ib study. *Journal of Clinical Oncology, 35*, 2117–2124.

Aron, M., Nguyen, M. M., Stein, R. J., & Gill, I. S. (2008). Impact of gender in renal cell carcinoma: An analysis of the SEER database. *European Urology, 54*, 133–140.

Atkins, M. B., Plimack, E. R., Puzanov, I., et al. (2016). Axitinib in combination with pembrolizumab in patients (pts) with advanced renal cell carcinoma (aRCC): Preliminary safety and efficacy results. *Annals of Oncology, 6*, 266, abstract 773PD.

Atkins, M. B., McDermott, D. F., Powles, T., et al. (2017). IMmotion150: A phase II trial in untreated metastatic renal cell carcinoma (mRCC) patients (pts) of atezolizumab (atezo) and bevacizumab (bev) vs and following atezo or sunitinib (sun) (abstract 4505). *2017 American Society of Clinical Oncology annual meeting.*

Balar, A. V., Galsky, M. D., Rosenberg, J. E., Powles, T., Petrylak, D. P., Bellmunt, J., Loriot, Y., Necchi, A., Hoffman-Censits, J., Perez-Gracia, J. L., Dawson, N. A., Van Der Heijden, M. S., Dreicer, R., Srinivas, S., Retz, M. M., Joseph, R. W., Drakaki, A., Vaishampayan, U. N., Sridhar, S. S., Quinn, D. I., Duran, I., Shaffer, D. R., Eigl, B. J., Grivas, P. D., Yu, E. Y., Li, S., Kadel, E. E., 3rd, Boyd, Z., Bourgon, R., Hegde, P. S., Mariathasan, S., Thastrom, A., Abidoye, O. O., Fine, G. D., Bajorin, D. F., & Group, I. M. S. (2017). Atezolizumab as first-line treatment in cisplatin-ineligible patients with locally advanced and metastatic urothelial carcinoma: A single-arm, multicentre, phase 2 trial. *Lancet, 389*, 67–76.

Bellmunt, J., De Wit, R., Vaughn, D. J., Fradet, Y., Lee, J. L., Fong, L., Vogelzang, N. J., Climent, M. A., Petrylak, D. P., Choueiri, T. K., Necchi, A., Gerritsen, W., Gurney, H., Quinn, D. I., Culine, S., Sternberg, C. N., Mai, Y., Poehlein, C. H., Perini, R. F., & Bajorin, D. F. (2017). Pembrolizumab as second-line therapy for advanced urothelial carcinoma. *New England Journal of Medicine, 376*, 1015–1026.

Brausi, M., Oddens, J., Sylvester, R., Bono, A., Van De Beek, C., Van Andel, G., Gontero, P., Turkeri, L., Marreaud, S., Collette, S., & Oosterlinck, W. (2014). Side effects of Bacillus Calmette-Guerin (BCG) in the treatment of intermediate- and high-risk Ta, T1 papillary carcinoma of the bladder: Results of the EORTC genito-urinary cancers group randomised phase 3 study comparing one-third dose with full dose and 1 year with 3 years of maintenance BCG. *European Urology, 65*, 69–76.

Cella, D., Grunwald, V., Nathan, P., Doan, J., Dastani, H., Taylor, F., Bennett, B., Derosa, M., Berry, S., Broglio, K., Berghorn, E., & Motzer, R. J. (2016). Quality of life in patients with advanced renal cell carcinoma given nivolumab versus everolimus in CheckMate 025: A randomised, open-label, phase 3 trial. *Lancet Oncology, 17*, 994–1003.

Choueiri, T. L. J., Oya, M., et al. (2017). First-line avelumab + axitinib therapy in patients (pts) with advanced renal cell carcinoma (aRCC): Results from a phase Ib trial (abstract 4504). *2017 American Society of Clinical Oncology annual meeting.*

Chow, W. H., & Devesa, S. S. (2008). Contemporary epidemiology of renal cell cancer. *The Cancer Journal, 14*, 288–301.

Chow, W. H., Devesa, S. S., Warren, J. L., & Fraumeni, J. F., Jr. (1999). Rising incidence of renal cell cancer in the United States. *JAMA, 281*, 1628–1631.

Dekernion, J. B., Sarna, G., Figlin, R., Lindner, A., & Smith, R. B. (1983). The treatment of renal cell carcinoma with human leukocyte alpha-interferon. *The Journal of Urology, 130*, 1063–1066.

Escudier, B., et al. (2017). LBA5-CheckMate 214: Efficacy and safety of nivolumab + ipilimumab (N+I) v sunitinib (S) for treatment-naïve advanced or metastatic renal cell carcinoma (mRCC), including IMDC risk and PD-L1 expression subgroups. ESMO 2017.

Escudier, B., Pluzanska, A., Koralewski, P., Ravaud, A., Bracarda, S., Szczylik, C., Chevreau, C., Filipek, M., Melichar, B., Bajetta, E., Gorbunova, V., Bay, J. O., Bodrogi, I., Jagiello-Gruszfeld, A., & Moore, N. (2007). Bevacizumab plus interferon alfa-2a for treatment of metastatic renal cell carcinoma: A randomised, double-blind phase III trial. *Lancet, 370*, 2103–2111.

Everson, T. C. (1964). Spontaneous regression of cancer. *Annals of the New York Academy of Sciences, 114*, 721–735.

Fisher, R. I., Rosenberg, S. A., & Fyfe, G. (2000). Long-term survival update for high-dose recombinant interleukin-2 in patients with renal cell carcinoma. *The Cancer Journal from Scientific American, 6*(Suppl 1), S55–S57.

Flanigan, R. C., Salmon, S. E., Blumenstein, B. A., Bearman, S. I., Roy, V., Mcgrath, P. C., Caton, J. R., Munshi, N., & Crawford, E. D. (2001). Nephrectomy followed by interferon alfa-2b compared with interferon alfa-2b alone for metastatic renal-cell cancer. *New England Journal of Medicine, 345*, 1655–1659.

Foot, N. C., Humphreys, G. A., & Whitmore, W. F. (1951). Renal tumors: Pathology and prognosis in 295 cases. *The Journal of Urology, 66*, 190–200.

Fuge, O., Vasdev, N., Allchorne, P., & Green, J. S. (2015). Immunotherapy for bladder cancer. *Research and Reports in Urology, 7*, 65–79.

Fyfe, G., Fisher, R. I., Rosenberg, S. A., Sznol, M., Parkinson, D. R., & Louie, A. C. (1995). Results of treatment of 255 patients with metastatic renal cell carcinoma who received high-dose recombinant interleukin-2 therapy. *Journal of Clinical Oncology, 13*, 688–696.

Gillett, M. D., Cheville, J. C., Karnes, R. J., Lohse, C. M., Kwon, E. D., Leibovich, B. C., Zincke, H., & Blute, M. L. (2005). Comparison of presentation and outcome for patients 18 to 40 and 60 to 70 years old with solid renal masses. *The Journal of Urology, 173*, 1893–1896.

Grawitz, P. (1883). Die sogenannten Lipome der Niere. *Arch Path Anat Physiol, 93*, 39–63.

Hallahan, J. D. (1959). Spontaneous remission of metastatic renal cell adenocarcinoma: A case report. *The Journal of Urology, 81*, 522–525.

Hammers, H. J., Plimack, E. R., Infante, J. R., Rini, B. I., Mcdermott, D. F., Lewis, L. D., Voss, M. H., Sharma, P., Pal, S. K., Razak, A. R. A., Kollmannsberger, C., Heng, D. Y. C., Spratlin, J., Mchenry, M. B., & Amin, A. (2017). Safety and efficacy of nivolumab in combination with ipilimumab in metastatic renal cell carcinoma: The checkMate 016 study. *Journal of Clinical Oncology*, JCO2016721985.

Jemal, A., Siegel, R., Ward, E., Hao, Y., Xu, J., & Thun, M. J. (2009). Cancer statistics, 2009. *CA: A Cancer Journal for Clinicians, 59*, 225–249.

Kamat, A. M., Hahn, N. M., Efstathiou, J. A., Lerner, S. P., Malmstrom, P. U., Choi, W., Guo, C. C., Lotan, Y., & Kassouf, W. (2016). Bladder cancer. *Lancet, 388*, 2796–2810.

Kamat, A. M., Bellmunt, J., Galsky, M. D., Konety, B. R., Lamm, D. L., Langham, D., Lee, C. T., Milowsky, M. I., O'Donnell, M. A., O'Donnell, P. H., Petrylak, D. P., Sharma, P., Skinner, E. C., Sonpavde, G., Taylor, J. A., 3rd, Abraham, P., & Rosenberg, J. E. (2017). Society for immunotherapy of cancer consensus statement on immunotherapy for the treatment of bladder carcinoma. *Journal for ImmunoTherapy of Cancer, 5*, 68.

Kane, C. J., Mallin, K., Ritchey, J., Cooperberg, M. R., & Carroll, P. R. (2008). Renal cell cancer stage migration: Analysis of the National Cancer Data Base. *Cancer, 113*, 78–83.

Levi, F., Ferlay, J., Galeone, C., Lucchini, F., Negri, E., Boyle, P., & La Vecchia, C. (2008). The changing pattern of kidney cancer incidence and mortality in Europe. *BJU International, 101*, 949–958.

Linn, J. F., Sesterhenn, I., Mostofi, F. K., & Schoenberg, M. (1998). The molecular characteristics of bladder cancer in young patients. *The Journal of Urology, 159*, 1493–1496.

Lynch, C. F., & Cohen, M. B. (1995). Urinary system. *Cancer, 75*, 316–329.

Massard, C., Gordon, M. S., Sharma, S., Rafii, S., Wainberg, Z. A., Luke, J., Curiel, T. J., Colon-Otero, G., Hamid, O., Sanborn, R. E., O'Donnell, P. H., Drakaki, A., Tan, W., Kurland, J. F., Rebelatto, M. C., Jin, X., Blake-Haskins, J. A., Gupta, A., & Segal, N. H. (2016). Safety and Efficacy of Durvalumab (MEDI4736), an anti-programmed cell death ligand-1 immune checkpoint inhibitor, in patients with advanced urothelial bladder cancer. *Journal of Clinical Oncology, 34*, 3119–3125.

Mcdermott, D. F., Sosman, J. A., Sznol, M., Massard, C., Gordon, M. S., Hamid, O., Powderly, J. D., Infante, J. R., Fasso, M., Wang, Y. V., Zou, W., Hegde, P. S., Fine, G. D., & Powles, T. (2016). Atezolizumab, an anti-programmed death-ligand 1 antibody, in metastatic renal cell carcinoma: Long-term safety, clinical activity, and immune correlates from a phase Ia study. *Journal of Clinical Oncology, 34*, 833–842.

Morales, A., Eidinger, D., & Bruce, A. W. (1976). Intracavitary Bacillus Calmette-Guerin in the treatment of superficial bladder tumors. *The Journal of Urology, 116*, 180–183.

Negrier, S., Escudier, B., Lasset, C., Douillard, J. Y., Savary, J., Chevreau, C., Ravaud, A., Mercatello, A., Peny, J., Mousseau, M., Philip, T., & Tursz, T. (1998). Recombinant human interleukin-2, recombinant human interferon alfa-2a, or both in metastatic renal-cell carcinoma. Groupe Francais d'Immunotherapie. *The New England Journal of Medicine, 338*, 1272–1278.

Oberling, C., Riviere, M., & Haguenau, F. (1960). Ultrastructure of the clear cells in renal carcinomas and its importance for the demonstration of their renal origin. *Nature, 186*, 402–403.

O'Donnell, P. H., Grivas, P., Balar, A. V., et al. (2017). Biomarker findings and mature clinical results from KEYNOTE-052: First-line pembrolizumab in cisplatin-ineligible advanced urothelial cancer (abstract 4502) *annual meeting American society of clinical oncology.*

Powles, T., Eder, J. P., Fine, G. D., Braiteh, F. S., Loriot, Y., Cruz, C., Bellmunt, J., Burris, H. A., Petrylak, D. P., Teng, S. L., Shen, X., Boyd, Z., Hegde, P. S., Chen, D. S., & Vogelzang, N. J. (2014). MPDL3280A (anti-PD-L1) treatment leads to clinical activity in metastatic bladder cancer. *Nature, 515*, 558–562.

Powles, T., O'Donnell, P. H., Massard, C., Arkenau, H. T., Friedlander, T. W., Hoimes, C. J., Lee, J. L., Ong, M., Sridhar, S. S., Vogelzang, N. J., Fishman, M. N., Zhang, J., Srinivas, S., Parikh, J., Antal, J., Jin, X., Gupta, A. K., Ben, Y., & Hahn, N. M. (2017). Efficacy and safety of durvalumab in locally advanced or metastatic urothelial carcinoma: Updated results from a phase 1/2 open-label study. *JAMA Oncology, 3*, e172411.

Rini, B. I., Halabi, S., Rosenberg, J. E., Stadler, W. M., Vaena, D. A., Ou, S. S., Archer, L., Atkins, J. N., Picus, J., Czaykowski, P., Dutcher, J., & Small, E. J. (2008). Bevacizumab plus interferon alfa compared with interferon alfa monotherapy in patients with metastatic renal cell carcinoma: CALGB 90206. *Journal of Clinical Oncology, 26*, 5422–5428.

Rini, B. I., Mcdermott, D. F., Hammers, H., Bro, W., Bukowski, R. M., Faba, B., Faba, J., Figlin, R. A., Hutson, T., Jonasch, E., Joseph, R. W., Leibovich, B. C., Olencki, T., Pantuck, A. J., Quinn, D. I., Seery, V., Voss, M. H., Wood, C. G., Wood, L. S., & Atkins, M. B. (2016). Society for immunotherapy of cancer consensus statement on immunotherapy for the treatment of renal cell carcinoma. *Journal for ImmunoTherapy of Cancer, 4*, 81.

Rosenberg, S. A., Yang, J. C., White, D. E., & Steinberg, S. M. (1998). Durability of complete responses in patients with metastatic cancer treated with high-dose interleukin-2: Identification of the antigens mediating response. *Annals Of Surgery, 228*, 307–319.

Rosenberg, J. E., Hoffman-Censits, J., Powles, T., Van Der Heijden, M. S., Balar, A. V., Necchi, A., Dawson, N., O'Donnell, P. H., Balmanoukian, A., Loriot, Y., Srinivas, S., Retz, M. M., Grivas,

P., Joseph, R. W., Galsky, M. D., Fleming, M. T., Petrylak, D. P., Perez-Gracia, J. L., Burris, H. A., Castellano, D., Canil, C., Bellmunt, J., Bajorin, D., Nickles, D., Bourgon, R., Frampton, G. M., Cui, N., Mariathasan, S., Abidoye, O., Fine, G. D., & Dreicer, R. (2016). Atezolizumab in patients with locally advanced and metastatic urothelial carcinoma who have progressed following treatment with platinum-based chemotherapy: A single-arm, multicentre, phase 2 trial. *The Lancet, 387*, 1909–1920.

Sanchez-Martin, F. M., Millan-Rodriguez, F., Urdaneta-Pignalosa, G., Rubio-Briones, J., & Villavicencio-Mavrich, H. (2008). Small renal masses: Incidental diagnosis, clinical symptoms, and prognostic factors. *Advances in Urology, 2008*, 310694.

Sharma, P., Callahan, M. K., Bono, P., Kim, J., Spiliopoulou, P., Calvo, E., Pillai, R. N., Ott, P. A., De Braud, F., Morse, M., Le, D. T., Jaeger, D., Chan, E., Harbison, C., Lin, C. S., Tschaika, M., Azrilevich, A., & Rosenberg, J. E. (2016). Nivolumab monotherapy in recurrent metastatic urothelial carcinoma (CheckMate 032): A multicentre, open-label, two-stage, multi-arm, phase 1/2 trial. *Lancet Oncology, 17*, 1590–1598.

Sharma, P., Retz, M., Siefker-Radtke, A., Baron, A., Necchi, A., Bedke, J., Plimack, E. R., Vaena, D., Grimm, M. O., Bracarda, S., Arranz, J. A., Pal, S., Ohyama, C., Saci, A., Qu, X., Lambert, A., Krishnan, S., Azrilevich, A., & Galsky, M. D. (2017). Nivolumab in metastatic urothelial carcinoma after platinum therapy (CheckMate 275): A multicentre, single-arm, phase 2 trial. *Lancet Oncology, 18*, 312–322.

Siegel, R. L., Miller, K. D., & Jemal, A. (2017). Cancer Statistics, 2017. *CA: A Cancer Journal for Clinicians, 67*, 7–30.

Smith, K. A. (1980). T-cell growth factor. *Immunology Reviews, 51*, 337–357.

Sylvester, R. J., Van Der Meijden, A. P., Witjes, J. A., & Kurth, K. (2005). Bacillus calmette-guerin versus chemotherapy for the intravesical treatment of patients with carcinoma in situ of the bladder: A meta-analysis of the published results of randomized clinical trials. *Journal Of Urology, 174*, 86–91; discussion 91-2.

Thompson, R. H., Ordonez, M. A., Iasonos, A., Secin, F. P., Guillonneau, B., Russo, P., & Touijer, K. (2008). Renal cell carcinoma in young and old patients–is there a difference? *Journal Of Urology, 180*, 1262–1266; discussion 1266.

Verhoest, G., Veillard, D., Guille, F., De La Taille, A., Salomon, L., Abbou, C. C., Valeri, A., Lechevallier, E., Descotes, J. L., Lang, H., Jacqmin, D., Tostain, J., Cindolo, L., Ficarra, V., Artibani, W., Schips, L., Zigeuner, R., Mulders, P. F., Mejean, A., & Patard, J. J. (2007). Relationship between age at diagnosis and clinicopathologic features of renal cell carcinoma. *European Urology, 51*, 1298–1304; discussion 1304-5.

Chapter 6
Next-Generation Immunotherapy in Lymphoma: Checkpoint Blockade, Chimeric Antigen Receptor T Cells, and Beyond

J.C. Villasboas

Contents

How Do Lymphomas Differ from Other Cancers?

The white cells that circulate in our blood are called leucocytes (from the Greek *leukos* for white) and constitute our primary line of defense against infections and cancer. In order to carry out their function, these highly specialized cells are required to identify foreign or abnormal molecules (non-self) and differentiate them from normal components of our system (self). When activated by the presence of non-self

J.C. Villasboas (✉)
Department of Medicine, Division of Hematology, Mayo Clinic, Rochester, MN, USA

© Springer International Publishing AG 2018
H. Dong, S.N. Markovic (eds.), *The Basics of Cancer Immunotherapy*,
https://doi.org/10.1007/978-3-319-70622-1_6

stimuli, these cells are programmed to trigger a cascade of biological events that will generate an inflammatory reaction responsible for eliminating the threat. This process is tightly regulated by a series of redundant biological mechanisms that will shut off the inflammatory response once the threat is eliminated and avoid excessive activation that could damage normal organs and systems in our body. These on/off systems allow our immunological defenses to function in a coordinated and self-regulated manner (Keir et al. 2008; Francisco et al. 2010; Bour-Jordan et al. 2011).

Many different groups of leukocytes exist in our body, each responsible for carrying out different but coordinated functions in order to maintain the health of our organism. Lymphocytes are a very special group of white cells and form the basis of our adaptive immune system (see Chap. 1 for a differentiation between innate and adaptive immune systems). Lymphocytes are able to specifically recognize a variety of foreign antigens, and once primed by the presence of these stimuli can transform into memory cells capable of rapidly recalling a specific immunological response. Just like virtually any cell in our body, lymphocytes are vulnerable to becoming corrupted and giving rise to cancer. We use the general term lymphoma to describe cancers generated from lymphocyte cells (Küppers 2005).

Patients afflicted by lymphomas typically present with tumoral masses in lymph nodes or other lymphoid tissues such as the tonsil and spleen. They may also have constitutional symptoms such as drenching night sweats, recurrent fever, and unintentional weight loss. At times, patients are diagnosed due to secondary lymphomatous involvement of other organs or structures such as the liver, bones, and skin. Lymphomas are grouped into two main categories: Hodgkin lymphomas (HLs) and non-Hodgkin lymphomas (NHLs), based on the appearance and characteristics of the cancerous cells when analyzed under the microscope. NHLs are typically further divided in two main categories (B-cell NHL and T-cell NHL) depending on the type of lymphocyte that gave rise to the cancer. Additional categorization can take place by dividing lymphomas into groups according to their behavior (indolent vs. aggressive) and other unique biological features. As a result, the World Health Organization (WHO) officially recognizes more than 70 distinct subtypes of lymphoma, and this number keeps growing as we gain more insight into the unique biology of each group (Swerdlow et al. 2016).

Lymphomas are a very special kind of cancer with unique characteristics that readily differentiate them from cancers arising in solid organs and tissues (such as the lung, intestine, breast, prostate, etc.). Similar to leukemias (cancer of the bone marrow), lymphomas are generally felt to represent systemic diseases. This means that lymphoma cells have direct access to the circulatory and lymphatic systems (an intrinsic property of lymphocytes from which they arise). As a result, localized treatment (i.e., surgery and/or radiotherapy) is generally ineffective to eradicate these cancers. There are notable exceptions to this rule, such as slow-growing (indolent) lymphomas localized to only one lymph node area that can be treated with radiation, but those are a minority of cases. For this reason, lymphomas and leukemias are often described as "liquid cancers" in contrast to "solid cancers" that arise in one organ or tissue and only access the bloodstream and lymphatic system in advanced stages. Systemic therapy (i.e., chemotherapy and/or immunotherapy) is therefore the mainstay of treatment for most patients with lymphoma, with localized therapy normally playing only an adjunctive role.

Another important distinction between lymphomas and solid cancers is that many lymphoma subtypes—typically the most aggressive ones—can be cured even when diagnosed at advanced stages (i.e., stage IV). Take the example of diffuse large B-cell lymphoma (DLBC), an aggressive B-cell NHL and the most common lymphoma subtype worldwide (Al-Hamadani et al. 2015; Smith et al. 2015; Kataoka et al. 2016b; Siegel et al. 2016). Patients diagnosed with stage IV DLBCL treated with chemoimmunotherapy have a chance of between 53% and 80% of being alive and free of disease 4 years after diagnosis (Sehn et al. 2007). This stands in sharp contrast to most patients diagnosed with metastatic (stage IV) cancer of the breast, lung, or colon in whom treatment is primarily palliative and intended to control the disease and alleviate symptoms. Despite our best efforts, most patients diagnosed with metastatic spread of a solid cancer are not curable although many advances have been made that allow us to control the disease.

In addition to their systemic nature, lymphoma cells originate from leucocytes, the same group of cells involved in defending our organisms from cancer itself. They can retain some of the properties and characteristics of normal leucocytes, which give them the ability to interact with and influence the normal immune system. Many lymphomas take advantage of this strategic position to alter, evade, or blunt the anti-cancer immune response, leaving the cancer process free to progress without effective opposition from the patient's immunological system. These characteristics are both the challenge and opportunity in this disease and make lymphomas suitable targets for immunotherapy. In this chapter we review the use of immunotherapy strategies in the management of lymphoma with a focus on recent advances including checkpoint inhibitors, chimeric antigen receptor (CAR) T-cell therapy, and novel immune-based treatment approaches.

The Enemy Within: How Lymphomas Escape Anti-Tumor Defenses Using Immunological Tools

The term tumor microenvironment (TME) has been loosely used to describe the non-cancerous cells and structures that surround cancer cells in the context of a tumor. The composition of that TME varies widely across the different types of cancer. Even within cancer of the same group—such as lymphomas—the composition of the TME can be very different, and this information is often helpful when differentiating amongst the many kinds of lymphomas. Take the example of classic HL (cHL) and DLBCL. When looking under the microscope at a tissue section from a lymph node affected by these lymphomas their appearance is quite different (Swerdlow 2008). DLBCL tumors are typically formed by numerous large cancerous cells with abnormal appearance intermixed with some inflammatory cells (part of the normal immune system). In contrast, in a lymph node affected by cHL you will see just a few cancerous cells (usually less than 10% of total cells) intermixed with a vast number of different inflammatory cells (Pileri et al. 2002). The obvious question is: how can these lymphomas thrive while surrounded by these cells and escape anti-cancer immune surveillance?

Part of the explanation lies in the fact that lymphoma cells are derived from lymphocytes and therefore have access to many of the resources available to the immune cells themselves. Using this strategic advantage, lymphoma cells may, for example, express on their surface proteins that facilitate their migration to other sites or secrete into their environment substances that stimulate cancer growth while inactivating normal immune cells. In many ways the behavior of lymphoma cells resembles that of a corrupted law enforcement agent who propagates negative behaviors using the resources meant to combat them. This intricate interplay between lymphoma cells and their microenvironment has been the focus of attention for many researchers in the field. While most details of this interaction remain to be elucidated, one thing is quite evident: the TME in lymphoma is far from a naïve bystander, as we will discuss in the next section (Gomez-Gelvez et al. 2016; Pizzi et al. 2016; Villasboas and Ansell 2016; Visser et al. 2016).

From Bystanders to Enablers: The Role of the Tumor Microenvironment in Supporting Lymphoma Growth

Lymphoma cells do not simply hide and escape from the immune system that surrounds them. In fact, these cancer cells actively manipulate their surroundings by inviting to their neighborhood specific types of immune cells that will support their growth (Liu et al. 2014; Vardhana and Younes 2016). At the same time, lymphoma cells will avoid or disable cells capable of effective tumor killing. Akin to the conductor, lymphoma cells are able to coordinate a complex malignant symphony that will alter the structure and function of normal immune cells. This results in a tumor microenvironment that not only promotes lymphoma growth but also facilitates escape from the immune system.

A good example of how lymphoma cells can influence the tumor microenvironment in their favor is the interaction between NHL and regulatory T (Treg) cells. Treg cells are a special family of T lymphocytes whose function is to monitor and control other lymphocytes in order to prevent excessive T-cell stimulation. Animal models and human disease states in which Tregs are dysfunctional or absent lead to autoimmunity—when the immune system fails to distinguish self from non-self and ends up attacking one's own body mistakenly (Dhaeze et al. 2015). The right amount of Tregs, therefore, is central to maintain the perfect immunological balance. What researchers have discovered is that lymphoma cells can skew that balance within their microenvironment by recruiting Tregs from the peripheral blood or inducing local Treg formation (Yang et al. 2007, 2009; Wang and Ke 2011). The result is an accumulation of Treg cells in the TME of lymphomas, which leads to a decrease in the function of effector immune cells.

Lymphoma cells are also able to influence their microenvironment by secreting soluble factors that lead to a state of immunological exhaustion. The phenomenon of immunological exhaustion was first characterized in the setting of chronic viral infections, where T lymphocytes that are chronically exposed to stimuli will lose their ability to react to it and effectively clear the infection. It was not until recently that a similar phenomenon was characterized in cancers including lymphomas (Yang et al. 2012, 2014, 2015). Many groups have now shown that lymphoma cells are able to secrete into their microenvironment (and into the bloodstream) substances that will lead to this state of immune tolerance, once again escaping anti-cancer surveillance (Yang et al. 2012; Xiu et al. 2015; Azzaoui et al. 2016). Exhausted T cells lose their ability to proliferate and are unable to produce the necessary effector molecules that normally lead to tumor clearance.

A third example of strategies used by lymphoma cells to evade the immune system is the hijacking of the immune checkpoint system (Dong et al. 2002; Wilcox et al. 2009; Kataoka et al. 2016a). These regulatory systems exist to prevent over-stimulation of T cells in the setting of an antigenic challenge. They act as the brakes on the immune system in such a way that a normal immunological response can be shut off after the threat has been cleared. One such system relies on the interaction between the programmed cell death receptor 1 (PD-1) and its ligands. In normal circumstances, when the PD-1 receptor (found on the surface of T lymphocytes) binds to a PD-1 ligand molecule (PD-L1 or PD-L2) found on the surface of other immune cells (such as macrophages, monocytes, dendritic cells) they receive a signal to shut off. Lymphoma cells can hijack this system by expressing PD-L1 on their surface, effectively blunting a tentative T-cell attack. Sometimes the expression of PD-L1 on the surface of lymphoma cells is driven by a genetic lesion (as is the case with cHL) or by the presence of a viral infection that contributes to lymphoma proliferation (as is the case with Epstein-Barr-infected lymphoma cells). Other times lymphoma cells will recruit to their neighborhood macrophages expressing PD-L1, creating the perfect niche for protection from the immune system (Carey et al. 2017).

The recruitment of Tregs and macrophages and the secretion of substances that lead to immunological exhaustion are just a few examples of resources used by lymphoma cells to alter their tumor microenvironment. This sets the perfect stage for the malignant process to progress but also generates opportunities for the development of cancer therapies targeting this very system.

First-Generation Immunotherapy in Lymphoma

The arsenal of drugs currently available to treat lymphoma already includes a number of therapies with an immunological basis. These treatments typically rely on the recognition of proteins on the surface of lymphoma cells using antibodies or related molecules. Antibody-drug conjugates have leveraged this property and work by tagging antibodies with toxic payloads in an attempt to deliver drugs in a precise manner to the interior of cancer cells. Many are now part of the standard-of-care for lymphoma patients, sometimes in combination with multi-drug chemotherapy regimens. Their efficacy relies on the early recognition that the specificity of the immune system can be used to target molecules present on cancer cells.

Monoclonal Antibodies

Rituximab is a monoclonal antibody (mAb) used routinely in the treatment of many B-cell NHLs. It recognizes a protein (CD20) found on the surface of normal B lymphocytes but also in most B-cell NHL cells (Maloney et al. 1997). This chimeric molecule (part human, part murine) was first introduced in the market in 1997 and became the first antibody approved by the US Food and Drug Administration (FDA) for the treatment of a human cancer. Several studies quickly followed to demonstrate the superior activity of rituximab in combination with chemotherapy compared to chemotherapy alone (Coiffier et al. 2002). Rituximab has altered the standard-of-care of B-cell NHL in such a way that the history of B-cell NHL treatment is typically divided in the pre-rituximab era and post-rituximab era owing to the remarkable improvement in clinical outcomes after the introduction of this drug. The impact of rituximab, however, extended far beyond the medical wards dedicated to the treatment of lymphoma patients. In fact, it inaugurated a new paradigm in cancer treatment usually referred to as chemoimmunotherapy.

Rituximab, and most monoclonal antibodies used in the treatment of cancer, are able of killing cancer cells using three main mechanisms: (i) complement-dependent cytotoxicity (CDC), (ii) antibody-dependent cellular toxicity (ADCC), and (iii) direct induction of apoptosis. In CDC, the antibody stuck to the surface of cancer cells serves as a tag that activates an immunological defense mechanism known as the complement system. This leads to a cascade of events mediated by components of this system found in our blood, which results in the formation of special proteins that puncture the membrane and kill cancer cells. In ADCC, the antibody is also used as an alert tag on the surface of the cancer cell, but this time the immunological attack is mediated by one of the effector cells of the normal immune system (i.e., macrophages, cytotoxic T cells). These cells will then produce toxic molecules that are discharged into or around the cancer cell, leading to apoptosis. Finally, when some monoclonal antibodies attach to proteins on the surface of a cancer cell they may turn on special signaling pathways inside the cells that directly leads to its death.

Driven by the success story of rituximab, many other monoclonal antibodies have now been developed for the treatment of lymphoma. Some of them target the same protein using molecules with slightly different properties. That is the case of obinutuzumab and ofatumumab, two humanized monoclonal antibodies recognizing CD20 that have been engineered to have increased cell-killing properties against CD20-expressing tumor cells (Mössner et al. 2010; Alduaij et al. 2011). Initial studies indicated that these drugs have activity in advanced lymphoma patients including some with previous exposure to rituximab-based therapy (Morschhauser et al. 2013; Ogura et al. 2013; Salles et al. 2013). Follow-up studies using these agents have had conflicting results and their exact role in the management of B-cell NHL is still to be elucidated. At this time the role of rituximab in standard-of-care of patients with CD20-expressing tumors has not been challenged by any of the newer CD20-targeting agents. In an attempt to reproduce the success of rituximab, antibodies recognizing other surface proteins were developed and tested in lymphoma. That is the case with epratuzumab, a mAb recognizing CD22 whose development was aborted despite an early signal of efficacy when combined with other chemoimmunotherapy regimens (Micallef et al. 2011). Alemtuzumab, a mAb targeting CD52, is another example of an immune-targeting drug available for the treatment of small lymphocytic lymphoma and some peripheral T-cell lymphomas (Dumitriu et al. 2016).

Antibody-Drug Conjugates and Radioimmunotherapy

A second wave of drug development followed the first ushered by the introduction of monoclonal antibodies into the care of cancer patients. This time the idea was to leverage the specificity of mAbs to achieve the long sought after effect of inducing toxicity on cancer cells while sparing the normal cells from untoward effects. This idea gave rise to two new concepts: antibody-drug conjugates (ADCs) and radioimmunotherapy.

ADCs are monoclonal antibodies charged with a toxic payload meant to be delivered specifically to cells expressing the protein target they recognize. Brentuximab vedotin (BV) is one such compound composed of a mAb recognizing CD30 loaded with monomethyl auristatin E (MMAE), a potent toxin that interferes with microtubule formation inside cells. MMAE is linked to the anti-CD30 antibody by a cleavable molecule that remains stable in the patient's blood but is digested once the compound enters the cancer cell. The effect is precise delivery of a toxic payload to the interior of the cancer cell along with relative sparing of normal tissue from unnecessary toxicity. cHL and anaplastic large T-cell lymphoma (ALTCL) are two cancers whose cells normally express CD30 on their surface. BV has now been tested and approved for the treatment of relapsed cHL and ALTCL (Pro et al. 2012; Younes et al. 2012). Isolated case reports and pre-clinical studies suggest that BV may have activity in other lymphomas expressing CD30 and therapy may be individualized beyond the standard FDA-labeled indications. Many other ADCs are currently under investigation using similar toxic payloads as BV (i.e., RG7593 (anti-CD22 plus auristatin) and SGN-CD19A (anti-CD19 plus auristatin)) or completely novel target-payload combinations (i.e. SAR3419 (anti-CD19 plus maytansine) and IMGN529 (anti-CD37 plus maytansine)).

Radioimmunotherapy (RIT) refers to the use of monoclonal antibodies to deliver radioactive molecules to the interior of cancer cells. Two such compounds were developed for the treatment of lymphoma patients: Yttrium-90 (Y-90)

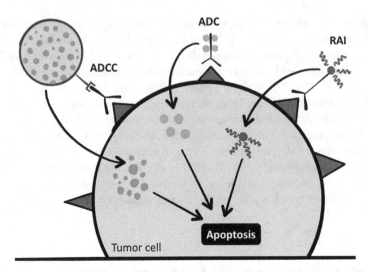

Fig. 6.1 Mechanisms of action of monoclonal antibodies (mAbs) and derivatives in lymphoma. Specific proteins (red triangle) are recognized by mAbs on the surface of the lymphoma cell. In antibody-dependent cellular cytotoxicity (ADCC) an effector immune cell is recruited and activated, releasing toxic granules on the interior of the tumor cell. Antibody drug conjugates (ADCs) attach to surface antigen and deliver a toxic payload that interferes with normal cellular functions. Radioimmunotherapy (RAI) compounds recognize surface antigens and deliver short-range ionizing radiation that leads to DNA damage. All processes have the end result of tumor cell death via apoptosis

ibritumomab tiuxetan (IDEC-Y2B8 or Zevalin®) and iodine-131 (I-131) tositumomab (Bexxar®). The drugs share a similar structure, with a mAb against CD20 tagged with a beta-emitting radioisotope. Studies in relapsed/refractory B-cell lymphomas demonstrated a clear efficacy signal with acceptable toxicity (Dillman 2002). Both drugs eventually received labeled indications for the treatment of B-cell NHL; however, Bexxar® was voluntarily withdrawn from the market by its manufacturer in 2014 due to low sales volume. Zevalin® remains available as a treatment option for B-cell NHL patients, but its widespread use has been limited by the logistics involved in the preparation and delivery of the drug, which requires involvement of nuclear medicine specialists in tertiary centers. A schematic overview of the mechanisms of action of monoclonal antibodies and its derivatives (ADC and RAI) is shown in Fig. 6.1.

Immunomodulatory Drugs (IMiDs)

Thalidomide analogs such as lenalidomide and pomalidomide are a group of agents defined loosely as immunomodulatory drugs (IMiDs), and demonstrate high activity against plasma cell neoplasms. These drugs seem to carry out their effect through multiple mechanisms and their efficacy is now being evaluated in patients with lymphoma. Many mechanisms of action of IMiDs have been postulated including: (i) direct anti-tumor activity via down-regulation of signaling pathways critical for cancer survival, (ii) changes in the configuration of the tumor microenvironment (TME) via interference with angiogenesis and adhesion molecules, (iii) enhancement of antibody activity via ADCC, (iv) halted expansion of immunosuppressive populations within the TME, such as Treg cells, and (v) increase in effector cell activity via co-stimulation of helper type 1 T cells (Th1), cytotoxic T cells, and natural killer (NK) cells.

IMiDs have been tested in both indolent and aggressive non-Hodgkin lymphomas. In mantle cell lymphoma, a rare type of B-cell NHL, lenalidomide demonstrated significant activity in patients with relapsed or refractory disease following standard chemoimmunotherapy (Habermann et al. 2009; Ahmadi et al. 2014). This led to the FDA approval of this drug in November of 2013 for patients with mantle cell lymphoma. Since then lenalidomide has been tested in other lymphoma subtypes and results thus far seem to indicate that the drug is active in other B-cell NHL subtypes, especially when combined with rituximab. A large multicenter randomized study comparing lenalidomide (L) + rituximab (R) with chemotherapy + rituximab in patients with untreated follicular lymphomas is ongoing. In parallel, a large multicenter phase II trial is evaluating the benefit of adding lenalidomide to standard chemoimmunotherapy in the first-line treatment of DLBCL, an aggressive B-cell NHL subtype. Both studies have completed accrual and the medical community anxiously awaits their results as they could promptly change the standard-of-care for lymphoma patients. Aside from mantle cell lymphoma, the use of lenalidomide is still considered experimental for most patients with NHL and cHL.

Next-Generation Immunotherapy in Lymphoma

As has been discussed up to this point, the use of immunological tools to treat patients with lymphoma is no novelty. Since 1997 oncologists have routinely used monoclonal antibodies to treat lymphoma and other cancers as standard practice. Building on this backbone inaugurated by rituximab, steady incremental progress was made by (i) the discovery of new antibodies, (ii) testing new antibody-chemotherapy combinations, and (iii) improvement in our ability to deliver these agents safely and with minimal side effects. As a result, the field of lymphoma therapy continued to move forward over the past 20 years. During this time, however, cancer immunotherapy continued to be studied in lymphoma and other cancers with erratic success. It was not until very recently when the field truly leapt forward with the introduction of the checkpoint inhibitors and chimeric antigen receptor (CAR) T cells. These new classes have revolutionized treatment for patients with many different types of cancer and represent a true breakthrough in our ability to harness the power of the immune system in the treatment of this disease. These next-generation immunotherapy drugs are re-shaping the way we think about and treat cancer, and herald the coming of a new era in the history of oncology. The following sections focus on the use of these newer immunotherapy agents in the context of the treatment of lymphoma.

Checkpoint Blockade

As explained earlier in the chapter, lymphoma cells have the ability to hijack natural regulatory systems known as immune checkpoints to de-activate T cells and protect themselves from an immune attack. Drugs such as ipilimumab, nivolumab, and pembrolizumab act on those immune checkpoints and interrupt the inhibitory signal coming from the malignant cells, effectively releasing T cells to carry out their immune attack. These drugs have now been tested in lymphoma patients and the following sections will detail their efficacy in this group.

CTLA-4 Inhibition

The cytotoxic T-lymphocyte antigen 4 (CTLA-4) receptor is expressed on the surface of T cells and works as a negative regulator of their function at the time of antigen presentation. If this receptor engages with the B7 molecule, expressed on the surface of the antigen-presenting cell (APC), it will give the T cell a signal to shut off its activity. Hence, the CTLA-4:B7 interaction is one of the immune checkpoints designed to control T cell overstimulation. Conversely, if the same B7 protein instead engages a CD28 molecule on the T cell it will produce a positive signal to stimulate T-cell function. Additionally, CTLA-4 is also expressed on Treg cells and stimulates their function such that the combination of effects caused by the CTLA-4:B7 interaction results in immune tolerance.

Ipilimumab, a monoclonal antibody that blocks CTLA-4, interferes with the interaction between CTLA-4 and B7 and is approved for the treatment of advanced melanoma. Three studies evaluated the activity of this agent in patients with advanced hematological malignancies including lymphomas.

The first study, published in 2009 by Bashey and colleagues, treated 29 patients with hematologic malignancies whose disease had recurred after an allogeneic stem cell transplant (Bashey et al. 2009). Patients received escalating doses of ipilimumab up to 3 mg/kg (single infusion). The primary purpose of the study was to evaluate the safety of this drug in this patient population. The drug was well tolerated and three patients with lymphoma experienced tumor shrinkage after treatment: two complete remissions in patients with cHL and one partial remission in a patient with mantle cell lymphoma. Albeit preliminarily, this study was the first to suggest that checkpoint inhibition was a safe and potentially efficacious strategy to treat patients with lymphoma.

Later that same year another study published by Ansell and colleagues evaluated the safety of ipilimumab in a cohort of patients with relapsed/refractory B-cell NHL lymphomas (Ansell et al. 2009). Patients in the initial cohort received 3 mg/kg induction followed by 1 mg/kg monthly maintenance (for a total of four doses) while the second-level cohort received 3 mg/kg monthly for 4 months. A total of 18 patients were treated and once again the drug demonstrated good tolerability. Two patients demonstrated a response: one patient with DLBCL who developed a complete response lasting more than 31 months and one patient with follicular lymphoma with a partial remission lasting 19 months. This small study confirmed the initial observation that ipilimumab, and possibly other checkpoint inhibitors, could be safely used in patients with lymphoma with the potential to induce long-lasting remissions.

An additional study published by Davids and colleagues in 2016 further explored the efficacy of ipilimumab in patients with hematologic malignancies whose disease had relapsed after an allogeneic transplant (Davids et al. 2016). Patients initially received ipilimumab at a dose of 3 mg/kg every 3 weeks but the dose level was subsequently escalated to 10 mg/kg every 3 weeks as no safety concerns were observed with the lower dose. A total of 28 patients with a variety of diagnoses were included in the study, of whom 11 had lymphoma. Immune-related adverse events and graft-versus-host disease developed in a significant proportion of patients, including one death. Amongst the patients with lymphoma, one had a partial response (cHL) and four had stable disease (three with cHL, one with a cutaneous T-cell NHL). No responses were seen in the patients who received the lower dose.

The knowledge generated collectively by these studies was sufficient to increase enthusiasm for the study of checkpoint inhibitors in patients with lymphoma. The experience with higher doses of ipilimumab suggested that efficacy could be increased but at the cost of more toxicity. Around this time, PD-1 blockers were emerging as a new class of checkpoint inhibitors in clinical trials in other malignancies demonstrating better safety and early evidence of higher efficacy. The development of additional studies using single-agent ipilimumab in lymphoid malignancies was quickly abandoned, although additional studies combining it with other immunotherapies are currently underway. At this time, ipilimumab use in lymphoma is considered experimental and not part of routine clinical practice.

PD-1 Blockade

The programmed cell death 1 (PD-1) pathway is another immune checkpoint mechanism of extreme importance in the regulation of T-cell function. When the PD-1 receptor, present on the surface of activated T cells, binds to one of its ligands (PD-L1 or PD-L2), it generates a signal that ultimately leads to the deactivation of these immune effector cells. When this regulatory mechanism is lacking or defective the result is the generation of auto-immunity and uncontrolled T-cell activity. Lymphoma cells are capable of taking advantage of this regulatory mechanism by either expressing the ligand on their surface or recruiting to their microenvironment other immune cells that will express those proteins. As a result, tumor-specific T cells are deactivated before they can carry out an anti-tumor attack. PD-1 inhibitors are monoclonal antibodies that attach to PD-1 and prevent it from receiving a signal from its ligands, thereby unleashing the T cells to carry out their anti-tumoral function effectively.

Two PD-1 inhibitors have been tested in lymphoma: nivolumab and pembrolizumab. Both drugs are monoclonal antibodies that block PD-1, and experience thus far seems to indicate that they have similar efficacy and safety, although no head-to-head comparisons exist. What seems strikingly different, however, is the degree of activity of these drugs in cHL compared to NHLs.

Nivolumab is a fully human antibody against the PD-1 receptor approved by the FDA on May 2016 for the treatment of relapsed or refractory cHL (r/r cHL) that has progressed after autologous stem cell transplant (ASCT) and post-transplantation brentuximab vedotin (BV). The approval was based on the results of two multi-center phase 2 trials (CheckMate 039 and CheckMate 205). In those studies, a combined total of 103 patients with r/r cHL received nivolumab 3 mg/kg IV every 2 weeks. A total of 65% of patients experienced a response, with 7% going to a complete remission. At least half of the patients who responded did so for at least 8.7 months, indicating that the effect was long-lasting. Treatment was well tolerated, and the most common side effects were fatigue, infusion reactions, and rash (Ansell et al. 2015).

Pembrolizumab is a humanized monoclonal antibody against PD-1 approved by the FDA on March 2017 for the treatment of r/r cHL after failure of at least three prior lines of therapy. The approval was based on the results of a multicenter phase 2 trial (Keynote-087) where 210 patients received pembrolizumab 200 mg IV every 3 weeks. A total of 69% of patients experienced a response, with 22.4% going into complete remission. Similarly, the drug was well tolerated and the most common side effects were fever, cough, and fatigue. Pembrolizumab is also approved for the treatment of pediatric cHL (Armand et al. 2016; Chen et al. 2017).

Patients with cHL seem to be disproportionally sensitive to PD-1 blockade therapy when compared to other cancers including NHL. This is notable not only by the number of cHL patients who respond to these drugs (60–70% in cHL compared to 15–20% in other cancers) but also by the duration of response (some cHL patients experiencing several months of response even after drug discontinuation). This can be at least partially explained by the genetic make-up of this disease where virtually all tumor cells overexpress PD-L1 and/or PD-L2. It has now been recognized that most cHLs do so because of a genetic lesion on chromosome 9 that results in over-production of the PD-1 ligands (Muenst et al. 2009; Green et al. 2010). Additionally, some cHL tumors are driven by infection with the Epstein-Barr virus, which can lead to PD-L1/2 overexpression by alternative pathways (Green et al. 2012). It is possible that additional mechanisms account for the sensitivity of PD-1 blockers in this disease and research in this field is ongoing. Exploring the unique sensitivity of cHL to PD-1 blockade several clinical trials are now underway investigating the role of adding these drugs in earlier phases of treatment.

While nivolumab and pembrolizumab were making headlines due to their remarkable activity in cHL, both drugs were tested in parallel for the treatment of advanced NHL. For this group of lymphomas, however, the activity with PD-1 blockade has been disappointingly small and short-lived (Lesokhin et al. 2016). In the initial studies of PD-1 blockade in NHL, less than 40% of patients experience some degree of response, all of them lasting just a short period. This observation led researchers in the field to hypothesize that the tumor microenvironment in NHL is skewed towards immune suppression to a degree that checkpoint blockade alone is not capable of reversing. As a result, many trials using combinatorial immunotherapy are currently underway or being developed for this patient population. At this time, the use of PD-1 inhibitors in NHL is considered experimental and not part of routine clinical practice.

Chimeric Antigen Receptor (CAR) T Cells

Another exciting breakthrough in the treatment of hematologic malignancies has been the recent development of the chimeric antigen receptor (CAR)-T cell technology. CAR-T cells are created by (i) removing T cells from a patient diagnosed with a cancer, (ii) isolating, activating, and genetically altering those cells in the laboratory, (iii) growing the genetically-engineered T cells in the laboratory, and (iv) re-introducing those cells to the patient after treatment with a low dose of chemotherapy. These modified T cells have special receptors on their surface and will be able to identify and kill tumor cells expressing a particular target protein with more proficiency than a normal T cell. One of the most transformative features of the CAR-T cell technology is that the "drug" is alive and therefore able to replicate inside the patient and expand their population for a system-wide anti-tumor attack. In August 2017, tisagenlecleucel (a CAR-T cell recognizing CD20) received FDA approval for the treatment of an aggressive form of leukemia (B-cell acute lymphoblastic leukemia) in patients up to the age of 25 years whose disease failed to response to standard treatment (Maude et al. 2014). The approval marked a historic moment with this drug being the first gene therapy to receive license for commercialization. Figure 6.2 is a schematic overview of the steps involved in CAR-T cell generation.

CAR-T cells are being actively studied in patients with lymphoma and most of the advance has been seen in aggressive B-cell NHL. Preliminary results of a study using axicabtagene ciloleucel (a CAR-T cell recognizing CD19) in aggressive B-cell NHL have now been released. Preliminary results on 101 patients with relapsed or refractory DLBCL treated with the CAR-T cell product in a multicenter phase II trial have been released. The drug demonstrated a high level of activity in this patient population, with 82% of patients showing response, 54% of them being complete remission. These results were presented at the annual meeting of the American Society of Clinical Oncology (ASCO) 2017 and not yet published. Most patients in the study had failed multiple lines of therapy including autologous stem cell transplant, and this degree of activity had never been seen in such refractory group. Investigators also showed that many of the responses were durable. Based on the results of this study, the manufacturer is seeking regulatory approval of this drug for patients with DLBCL and a decision is expected no later than early 2018. Additional studies evaluating the use of CAR-T in other patients with NHL and cHL are underway.

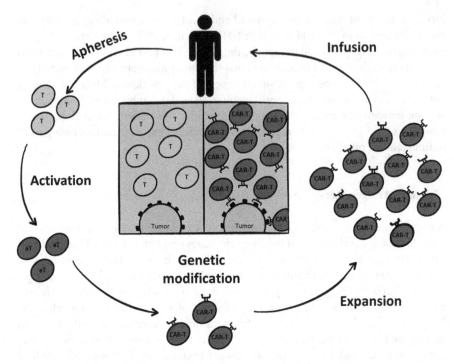

Fig. 6.2 Schematic of chimeric antigen receptor (CAR)-T cell generation. T cells (T) are removed (apheresis) from the peripheral blood of a patients diagnosed with lymphoma. In the laboratory, these cells are activated (aT) and genetically modified to express an engineered receptor on their surface (CAR-T). After expansion, CAR-T cells are administered to the patient (infusion) and can now recognize the kill tumor cells

Novel Immunological Targets and Dual Immunomodulation

The contrasting activity of PD-1 blockade between patients with cHL and NHL has been the focus of interest for many researchers in the field. As new discoveries are made, the role of the tumor microenvironment (TME) as a master regulator of lymphoma progression is emerging as a recurrent theme. In the case of NHL, it seems that the TME not only deactivates competent T cells (via immune checkpoint pathways) but also actively drives T cell to exhaustion through soluble molecules and inhibitory cells (Treg cells, myeloid-derived suppressor cells, etc.). The degree of suppression that results is postulated to be beyond rescue by PD-1 blockade alone. Additional molecules leading to immunosuppression (i.e., TIM-3, LAG-3) have also been identified in the lymphoma TME, and drugs blocking their activity are being tested.

The next frontier of lymphoma immunotherapy will be testing whether dual immunomodulation can reverse effector cells from the suppressive microenvironment that surrounds malignant cells. One proposed strategy is to release T cells from checkpoint-mediated immunosuppression (with a PD-1 inhibitor) while at the same time igniting T-cell activity with antibodies that stimulate their function (i.e., varlilumab or CDX-1127) in order to rescue them from exhaustion. If the T cell were a car, this strategy would be analogous to taking the foot off its break (PD-1 blockade) while hitting the gas pedal (CD-27 stimulation) so it can go after and kill cancer cells. Studies using this—and other—drug combinations are being developed or are underway.

The Future of Lymphoma Immunotherapy

The recent advances in the field of cancer immunotherapy leave no doubt that this treatment strategy is here to stay. New drugs and technologies are arriving with such disruptive and innovative power that they will forever transform the way we treat—and think about—cancer. The question to ask is not if but how we will incorporate these advances into the standard treatment of patients with lymphoma. We cannot forget that, in many cases, lymphomas can be cured with the treatments currently available. It is also true that sometimes treatments may cause long-term side effects in survivors. One of the challenges will be incorporating these new drugs into the treatment algorithm so that cure rates can increase while curtailing side effects. Another important issue that invariably accompanies these new drugs is the high cost. As immunotherapy drugs become more widely used, effort needs to be made to study their cost-effectiveness from both an individual and a health system perspective. From the perspective of the oncologists, treatment individualization will be ever more important to identify the best selection, sequence, and duration of treatment for each and every patient sitting in front of them. We are living through very exciting times in rapid transformation and one cannot avoid to hope we are moving towards the ultimate goal of one day curing every patient with lymphoma—one T cell at a time.

References

Ahmadi, T., Chong, E. A., Gordon, A., Aqui, N. A., Nasta, S. D., Svoboda, J., Mato, A. R., & Schuster, S. J. (2014). Combined lenalidomide, low-dose dexamethasone, and rituximab achieves durable responses in rituximab-resistant indolent and mantle cell lymphomas. *Cancer, 120*(2), 222–228. https://doi.org/10.1002/cncr.28405.

Alduaij, W., Ivanov, A., Honeychurch, J., Cheadle, E. J., Potluri, S., Lim, S. H., Shimada, K., Chan, C. H. T., Tutt, A., Beers, S. A., Glennie, M. J., Cragg, M. S., & Illidge, T. M. (2011). Novel type II anti-CD20 monoclonal antibody (GA101) evokes homotypic adhesion and actin-dependent, lysosome-mediated cell death in B-cell malignancies. *Blood, 117*(17), 4519–4529. https://doi.org/10.1182/blood-2010-07-296913.

Al-Hamadani, M., Habermann, T. M., Cerhan, J. R., Macon, W. R., Maurer, M. J., & Go, R. S. (2015). Non-Hodgkin lymphoma subtype distribution, geodemographic patterns, and survival in the US: A longitudinal analysis of the National Cancer Data Base from 1998 to 2011. *American Journal of Hematology, 90*(9), 790–795. https://doi.org/10.1002/ajh.24086.

Ansell, S. M., Hurvitz, S. A., Koenig, P. A., LaPlant, B. R., Kabat, B. F., Fernando, D., Habermann, T. M., Inwards, D. J., Verma, M., Yamada, R., Erlichman, C., Lowy, I., & Timmerman, J. M. (2009). Phase I study of ipilimumab, an anti-CTLA-4 monoclonal antibody, in patients with relapsed and refractory B-cell non-Hodgkin lymphoma. *Clinical Cancer Research, 15*(20), 6446–6453. https://doi.org/10.1158/1078-0432.CCR-09-1339.

Ansell, S. M., Lesokhin, A. M., Borrello, I., Halwani, A., Scott, E. C., Gutierrez, M., Schuster, S. J., Millenson, M. M., Cattry, D., Freeman, G. J., Rodig, S. J., Chapuy, B., Ligon, A. H., Zhu, L., Grosso, J. F., Kim, S. Y., Timmerman, J. M., Shipp, M. A., & Armand, P. (2015). PD-1 blockade with nivolumab in relapsed or refractory Hodgkin's lymphoma. *The New England Journal of Medicine, 372*(4), 311–319. https://doi.org/10.1056/NEJMoa1411087.

Armand, P., Shipp, M. A., Ribrag, V., Michot, J. M., Zinzani, P. L., Kuruvilla, J., Snyder, E. S., Ricart, A. D., Balakumaran, A., Rose, S., & Moskowitz, C. H. (2016). Programmed death-1 blockade with pembrolizumab in patients with classical hodgkin lymphoma after brentuximab vedotin failure. *Journal of Clinical Oncology: Official Journal of the American Society of Clinical Oncology.* https://doi.org/10.1200/JCO.2016.67.3467.

Azzaoui, I., Uhel, F., Rossille, D., Pangault, C., Dulong, J., Le Priol, J., Lamy, T., Houot, R., Le Gouill, S., Cartron, G., Godmer, P., Bouabdallah, K., Milpied, N., Damaj, G., Tarte, K., Fest, T., & Roussel, M. (2016). T-cell defect in diffuse large B-cell lymphomas involves expansion of myeloid derived suppressor cells expressing IL-10, PD-L1 and S100A12. *Blood*, blood-2015-08-662783. https://doi.org/10.1182/blood-2015-08-662783.

Bashey, A., Medina, B., Corringham, S., Pasek, M., Carrier, E., Vrooman, L., Lowy, I., Solomon, S. R., Morris, L. E., Holland, H. K., Mason, J. R., Alyea, E. P., Soiffer, R. J., & Ball, E. D. (2009). CTLA4 blockade with ipilimumab to treat relapse of malignancy after allogeneic hematopoietic cell transplantation. *Blood, 113*(7), 1581–1588. https://doi.org/10.1182/blood-2008-07-168468.

Bour-Jordan, H., Esensten, J. H., Martinez-Llordella, M., Penaranda, C., Stumpf, M., & Bluestone, J. A. (2011). Intrinsic and extrinsic control of peripheral T-cell tolerance by costimulatory molecules of the CD28/ B7 family. *Immunological Reviews, 241*(1), 180–205. https://doi.org/10.1111/j.1600-065X.2011.01011.x.

Carey, C. D., Gusenleitner, D., Lipschitz, M., Roemer, M. G. M., Stack, E. C., Gjini, E., Hu, X., Redd, R., Freeman, G. J., Neuberg, D., Hodi, F. S., Liu, X. S., Shipp, M. A., & Rodig, S. J. (2017). Topological analysis reveals a PD-L1 associated microenvironmental niche for Reed-Sternberg cells in Hodgkin lymphoma. *Blood, Elsevier Inc., 46*(1), 148–161. https://doi.org/10.1182/blood-2017-03-770719.

Chen, R., Zinzani, P. L., Fanale, M. A., Armand, P., Johnson, N. A., Brice, P., Radford, J., Ribrag, V., Molin, D., Vassilakopoulos, T. P., Tomita, A., von Tresckow, B., Shipp, M. A., Zhang, Y., Ricart, A. D., Balakumaran, A., Moskowitz, C. H., & KEYNOTE-087. (2017). Phase II study of the efficacy and safety of pembrolizumab for relapsed/refractory classic hodgkin lymphoma. *Journal of Clinical Oncology: Official Journal of the American Society of Clinical Oncology, 1*, JCO2016721316. https://doi.org/10.1200/JCO.2016.72.1316.

Coiffier, B., Lepage, E., Briere, J., Herbrecht, R., Tilly, H., Bouabdallah, R., Morel, P., Van Den Neste, E., Salles, G., Gaulard, P., Reyes, F., Lederlin, P., & Gisselbrecht, C. (2002). CHOP chemotherapy plus rituximab compared with CHOP alone in elderly patients with diffuse large-B-cell lymphoma. *The New England journal of medicine.* https://doi.org/10.1056/NEJMoa011795.

Davids, M. S., Kim, H. T., Bachireddy, P., Costello, C., Liguori, R., Savell, A., Lukez, A. P., Avigan, D., Chen, Y. B., McSweeney, P., LeBoeuf, N. R., Rooney, M. S., Bowden, M., Zhou, C. W., Granter, S. R., Hornick, J. L., Rodig, S. J., Hirakawa, M., Severgnini, M., Hodi, F. S., Wu, C. J., Ho, V. T., Cutler, C., Koreth, J., Alyea, E. P., Antin, J. H., Armand, P., Streicher, H., Ball, E. D., Ritz, J., Bashey, A., Soiffer, R. J., & Leukemia and Lymphoma Society Blood Cancer Research Partnership. (2016). Ipilimumab for patients with relapse after allogeneic transplantation. *The New England Journal of Medicine, 375*(2), 143–153. https://doi.org/10.1056/NEJMoa1601202.

Dhaeze, T., Stinissen, P., Liston, A., & Hellings, N. (2015). Humoral autoimmunity: A failure of regulatory T cells? *Autoimmunity Reviews*. Elsevier B.V, *14*(8), 735–741. https://doi. org/10.1016/j.autrev.2015.04.006.

Dillman, R. O. (2002). Radiolabeled anti-CD20 monoclonal antibodies for the treatment of B-cell lymphoma. *Journal of Clinical Oncology: Official Journal of the American Society of Clinical Oncology, 20*(16), 3545–3557. https://doi.org/10.1200/JCO.2002.02.126.

Dong, H., Strome, S. E., Salomao, D. R., Tamura, H., Hirano, F., Flies, D. B., Roche, P. C., Lu, J., Zhu, G., Tamada, K., Lennon, V. A., Celis, E., & Chen, L. (2002). Tumor-associated B7-H1 promotes T-cell apoptosis: A potential mechanism of immune evasion. *Nature medicine, 8*(8), 793–800. https://doi.org/10.1038/nm730.

Dumitriu, B., Ito, S., Feng, X., Stephens, N., Yunce, M., Kajigaya, S., Melenhorst, J. J., Rios, O., Scheinberg, P., Chinian, F., Keyvanfar, K., Battiwalla, M., Wu, C. O., Maric, I., Xi, L., Raffeld, M., Muranski, P., Townsley, D. M., Young, N. S., Barrett, A. J., & Scheinberg, P. (2016). Alemtuzumab in T-cell large granular lymphocytic leukaemia: Interim results from a single-arm, open-label, phase 2 study. *The Lancet. Haematology*, Elsevier Ltd, *3*(1), e22–e29. https://doi.org/10.1016/S2352-3026(15)00227-6.

Francisco, L. M., Sage, P. T., & Sharpe, A. H. (2010). The PD-1 pathway in tolerance and autoimmunity. *Immunological Reviews*, 219–242. https://doi.org/10.1111/j.1600-065X.2010.00923.x.

Gomez-Gelvez, J. C., Salama, M. E., Perkins, S. L., Leavitt, M., & Inamdar, K. V. (2016). Prognostic impact of tumor microenvironment in diffuse large B-Cell lymphoma uniformly treated with R-CHOP chemotherapy. *American Journal of Clinical Pathology, 145*(4), 514–523. https://doi.org/10.1093/ajcp/aqw034.

Green, M. R., Monti, S., Rodig, S. J., Juszczynski, P., Currie, T., O'Donnell, E., Chapuy, B., Takeyama, K., Neuberg, D., Golub, T. R., Kutok, J. L., & Shipp, M. A. (2010). Integrative analysis reveals selective 9p24.1 amplification, increased PD-1 ligand expression, and further induction via JAK2 in nodular sclerosing Hodgkin lymphoma and primary mediastinal large B-cell lymphoma. *Blood, 116*(17), 3268–3277. https://doi.org/10.1182/blood-2010-05-282780.

Green, M. R., Rodig, S., Juszczynski, P., Ouyang, J., Sinha, P., O'Donnell, E., Neuberg, D., & Shipp, M. A. (2012). Constitutive AP-1 activity and EBV infection induce PD-l1 in Hodgkin lymphomas and posttransplant lymphoproliferative disorders: Implications for targeted therapy. *Clinical Cancer Research, 18*(6), 1611–1618. https://doi.org/10.1158/1078-0432. CCR-11-1942.

Habermann, T. M., Lossos, I. S., Justice, G., Vose, J. M., Wiernik, P. H., McBride, K., Wride, K., Ervin-Haynes, A., Takeshita, K., Pietronigro, D., Zeldis, J. B., & Tuscano, J. M. (2009). Lenalidomide oral monotherapy produces a high response rate in patients with relapsed or refractory mantle cell lymphoma. *British Journal of Haematology, 145*(3), 344–349. https:// doi.org/10.1111/j.1365-2141.2009.07626.x.

Kataoka, K., Shiraishi, Y., Takeda, Y., Sakata, S., Matsumoto, M., Nagano, S., Maeda, T., Nagata, Y., Kitanaka, A., Mizuno, S., Tanaka, H., Chiba, K., Ito, S., Watatani, Y., Kakiuchi, N., Suzuki, H., Yoshizato, T., Yoshida, K., Sanada, M., Itonaga, H., Imaizumi, Y., Totoki, Y., Munakata, W., Nakamura, H., Hama, N., Shide, K., Kubuki, Y., Hidaka, T., Kameda, T., Masuda, K., Minato, N., Kashiwase, K., Izutsu, K., Takaori-Kondo, A., Miyazaki, Y., Takahashi, S., Shibata, T., Kawamoto, H., Akatsuka, Y., Shimoda, K., Takeuchi, K., Seya, T., Miyano, S., & Ogawa, S. (2016a). Aberrant PD-L1 expression through 3'-UTR disruption in multiple cancers. *Nature*, Nature Publishing Group, *534*(7607), 402–6. https://doi.org/10.1038/nature18294.

Kataoka, K., Shiraishi, Y., Takeda, Y., Sakata, S., Matsumoto, M., Nagano, S., Maeda, T., Nagata, Y., Kitanaka, A., Mizuno, S., Tanaka, H., Chiba, K., Ito, S., Watatani, Y., Kakiuchi, N., Suzuki, H., Yoshizato, T., Yoshida, K., Sanada, M., Itonaga, H., Imaizumi, Y., Totoki, Y., Munakata, W., Nakamura, H., Hama, N., Shide, K., Kubuki, Y., Hidaka, T., Kameda, T., Masuda, K., Minato, N., Kashiwase, K., Izutsu, K., Takaori-Kondo, A., Miyazaki, Y., Takahashi, S., Shibata, T., Kawamoto, H., Akatsuka, Y., Shimoda, K., Takeuchi, K., Seya, T., Miyano, S., & Ogawa, S. (2016b). Non-hodgkin lymphoma in the developing world: review of 4539 cases from the international non-hodgkin lymphoma classification project. *Nature, 534*(7607), 402–406. https:// doi.org/10.3324/haematol.2016.148809.

Keir, M. E., Butte, M. J., Freeman, G. J., & Sharpe, A. H. (2008). PD-1 and its ligands in tolerance and immunity. *Annual Review of Immunology, 26,* 677–704. https://doi.org/10.1146/annurev. immunol.26.021607.090331.

Küppers, R. (2005). Mechanisms of B-cell lymphoma pathogenesis. *Nature reviews. Cancer, 5*(4), 251–262. https://doi.org/10.1038/nrc1589.

Lesokhin, A. M., Ansell, S. M., Armand, P., Scott, E. C., Halwani, A., Gutierrez, M., Millenson, M. M., Cohen, A. D., Schuster, S. J., Lebovic, D., Dhodapkar, M., Avigan, D., Chapuy, B., Ligon, A. H., Freeman, G. J., Rodig, S. J., Cattry, D., Zhu, L., Grosso, J. F., Bradley Garelik, M. B., Shipp, M. A., Borrello, I., & Timmerman, J. (2016). Nivolumab in patients with relapsed or refractory hematologic malignancy: Preliminary results of a phase Ib study. *Journal of Clinical Oncology: Official Journal of the American Society of Clinical Oncology, 34*(23), 2698–2704. https://doi.org/10.1200/JCO.2015.65.9789.

Liu, Y., Sattarzadeh, A., Diepstra, A., Visser, L., & van den Berg, A. (2014). The microenvironment in classical Hodgkin lymphoma: An actively shaped and essential tumor component. *Seminars in Cancer Biology, 24,* 15–22. https://doi.org/10.1016/j.semcancer.2013.07.002.

Maloney, D. G., Grillo-López, A. J., White, C. A., Bodkin, D., Schilder, R. J., Neidhart, J. A., Janakiraman, N., Foon, K. A., Liles, T. M., Dallaire, B. K., Wey, K., Royston, I., Davis, T., & Levy, R. (1997). IDEC-C2B8 (Rituximab) anti-CD20 monoclonal antibody therapy in patients with relapsed low-grade non-Hodgkin's lymphoma. *Blood, 90*(6), 2188–2195.

Maude, S. L., Frey, N., Shaw, P. A., Aplenc, R., Barrett, D. M., Bunin, N. J., Chew, A., Gonzalez, V. E., Zheng, Z., Lacey, S. F., Mahnke, Y. D., Melenhorst, J. J., Rheingold, S. R., Shen, A., Teachey, D. T., Levine, B. L., June, C. H., Porter, D. L., & Grupp, S. A. (2014). Chimeric antigen receptor T cells for sustained remissions in leukemia. *The New England Journal of Medicine, 371*(16), 1507–1517. https://doi.org/10.1056/NEJMoa1407222.

Micallef, I. N. M., Maurer, M. J., Wiseman, G. A., Nikcevich, D. A., Kurtin, P. J., Cannon, M. W., Perez, D. G., Soori, G. S., Link, B. K., Habermann, T. M., & Witzig, T. E. (2011). Epratuzumab with rituximab, cyclophosphamide, doxorubicin, vincristine, and prednisone chemotherapy in patients with previously untreated diffuse large B-cell lymphoma. *Blood, 118*(15), 4053–4061. https://doi.org/10.1182/blood-2011-02-336990.

Morschhauser, F. A., Cartron, G., Thieblemont, C., Solal-Céligny, P., Haioun, C., Bouabdallah, R., Feugier, P., Bouabdallah, K., Asikanius, E., Lei, G., Wenger, M., Wassner-Fritsch, E., & Salles, G. A. (2013). Obinutuzumab (GA101) monotherapy in relapsed/refractory diffuse large b-cell lymphoma or mantle cell lymphoma: results from the phase II GAUGUIN study. *Journal of Clinical Oncology: Official Journal of the American Society of Clinical Oncology, 31*(23), 2912–2919. https://doi.org/10.1200/JCO.2012.46.9585.

Mössner, E., Brünker, P., Moser, S., Püntener, U., Schmidt, C., Herter, S., Grau, R., Gerdes, C., Nopora, A., Van Puijenbroek, E., Ferrara, C., Sondermann, P., Jäger, C., Strein, P., Fertig, G., Friess, T., Schüll, C., Bauer, S., Dal Porto, J., Del Nagro, C., Dabbagh, K., Dyer, M. J. S., Poppema, S., Klein, C., & Umaña, P. (2010). Increasing the efficacy of CD20 antibody therapy through the engineering of a new type II anti-CD20 antibody with enhanced direct and immune effector cell – mediated B-cell cytotoxicity. *Blood, 115*(22), 4393–4402. https://doi.org/10.1182/blood-2009-06-225979.

Muenst, S., Hoeller, S., Dirnhofer, S., & Tzankov, A. (2009). Increased programmed death-1+ tumor-infiltrating lymphocytes in classical Hodgkin lymphoma substantiate reduced overall survival. *Human pathology,* Elsevier Inc, *40*(12), 1715–1722. https://doi.org/10.1016/j. humpath.2009.03.025.

Ogura, M., Tobinai, K., Hatake, K., Uchida, T., Suzuki, T., Kobayashi, Y., Mori, M., Terui, Y., Yokoyama, M., & Hotta, T. (2013). Phase I study of obinutuzumab (GA101) in Japanese patients with relapsed or refractory B-cell non-Hodgkin lymphoma. *Cancer Science, 104*(1), 105–110. https://doi.org/10.1111/cas.12040.

Pileri, S. A., Ascani, S., Leoncini, L., Sabattini, E., Zinzani, P. L., Piccaluga, P. P., Pileri, A., Giunti, M., Falini, B., Bolis, G. B., & Stein, H. (2002). Hodgkin's lymphoma: The pathologist's viewpoint. *Journal of clinical pathology, 55,* 162–176. https://doi.org/10.1136/jcp.55.3.162.

Pizzi, M., Boi, M., Bertoni, F., & Inghirami, G. (2016). Emerging therapies provide new opportunities to reshape the multifaceted interactions between the immune system and lymphoma cells. *Leukemia*, Nature Publishing Group, *30*(9), 1805–1815. https://doi.org/10.1038/leu.2016.161.

Pro, B., Advani, R., Brice, P., Bartlett, N. L., Rosenblatt, J. D., Illidge, T., Matous, J., Ramchandren, R., Fanale, M., Connors, J. M., Yang, Y., Sievers, E. L., Kennedy, D. A., & Shustov, A. (2012). Brentuximab vedotin (SGN-35) in patients with relapsed or refractory systemic anaplastic large-cell lymphoma: Results of a phase II study. *Journal of Clinical Oncology, 30*(18), 2190–2196. https://doi.org/10.1200/JCO.2011.38.0402.

Salles, G. A., Morschhauser, F., Solal-Céligny, P., Thieblemont, C., Lamy, T., Tilly, H., Gyan, E., Lei, G., Wenger, M., Wassner-Fritsch, E., & Cartron, G. (2013). Obinutuzumab (GA101) in patients with relapsed/refractory indolent non-Hodgkin lymphoma: results from the phase II GAUGUIN study. *Journal of Clinical Oncology: Official Journal of the American Society of Clinical Oncology, 31*(23), 2920–2926. https://doi.org/10.1200/JCO.2012.46.9718.

Sehn, L. H., Berry, B., Chhanabhai, M., Fitzgerald, C., Gill, K., Hoskins, P., Klasa, R., Savage, K. J., Shenkier, T., Sutherland, J., Gascoyne, R. D., & Connors, J. M. (2007). The revised international prognostic index (R-IPI) is a better predictor of outcome than the standard IPI for patients with diffuse large B-cell lymphoma treated with R-CHOP. *Blood, 109*(5), 1857–1861. https://doi.org/10.1182/blood-2006-08-038257.

Siegel, R. L., Miller, K. D., & Jemal, A. (2016). Cancer statistics, 2016. *CA: A Cancer Journal for Clinicians, 66*(1), 7–30. https://doi.org/10.3322/caac.21332.

Smith, A., Crouch, S., Lax, S., Li, J., Painter, D., Howell, D., Patmore, R., Jack, A., & Roman, E. (2015). Lymphoma incidence, survival and prevalence 2004-2014: Sub-type analyses from the UK's Haematological malignancy research network. *British Journal of Cancer, 112*(9), 1575–1584. https://doi.org/10.1038/bjc.2015.94.

Swerdlow, S. H. (2008). *WHO classification of tumours of haematopoietic and lymphoid tissues* (4th ed.). Lyon, France: International Agency for Research on Cancer.

Swerdlow, S. H., Campo, E., Pileri, S. A., Harris, N. L., Stein, H., Siebert, R., Advani, R., Ghielmini, M., Salles, G. A., Zelenetz, A. D., & Jaffe, E. S. (2016). The 2016 revision of the World Health Organization classification of lymphoid neoplasms. *Blood, 127*(20), 2375–2390. https://doi.org/10.1182/blood-2016-01-643569.

Vardhana, S., & Younes, A. (2016). The immune microenvironment in Hodgkin lymphoma: T cells, B cells, and immune checkpoints. *Haematologica, 101*(7), 794–802. https://doi.org/10.3324/haematol.2015.132761.

Villasboas, J. C., & Ansell, S. (2016). Glancing at the complex biology of T-cells through the microenvironment of hodgkin lymphoma. *Leukemia & lymphoma*, 1–3. https://doi.org/10.1080/10428194.2016.1248966.

Visser, L., Wu, R., Rutgers, B., Diepstra, A., & van den Berg, A. (2016). Characterization of the microenvironment of nodular lymphocyte predominant hodgkin lymphoma. *International journal of molecular sciences, 17*(12), 2127. https://doi.org/10.3390/ijms17122127.

Wang, J., & Ke, X. Y. (2011). The four types of Tregs in malignant lymphomas. *Journal of hematology & oncology, 4*(1), 50. https://doi.org/10.1186/1756-8722-4-50.

Wilcox, R. A., Feldman, A. L., Wada, D. A., Yang, Z. Z., Comfere, N. I., Dong, H., Kwon, E. D., Novak, A. J., Markovic, S. N., Pittelkow, M. R., Witzig, T. E., & Ansell, S. M. (2009). B7-H1 (PD-L1, CD274) suppresses host immunity in T-cell lymphoproliferative disorders. *Blood, 114*(10), 2149–2158. https://doi.org/10.1182/blood-2009-04-216671.

Xiu, B., Lin, Y., Grote, D. M., Ziesmer, S. C., Gustafson, M. P., Maas, M. L., Zhang, Z., Dietz, A. B., Porrata, L. F., Novak, A. J., Liang, A.-B., Yang, Z.-Z., & Ansell, S. M. (2015). IL-10 induces the development of immunosuppressive CD14(+)HLA-DR(low/-) monocytes in B-cell non-Hodgkin lymphoma. *Blood Cancer Journal, 5*(March), e328. https://doi.org/10.1038/bcj.2015.56.

Yang, Z. Z., Novak, A. J., Ziesmer, S. C., Witzig, T. E., & Ansell, S. M. (2007). CD70+ non-Hodgkin lymphoma B cells induce Foxp3 expression and regulatory function in intratumoral CD4+CD25- T cells. *Blood, 110*(7), 2537–2544. https://doi.org/10.1182/blood-2007-03-082578.

Yang, Z. Z., Novak, A. J., Ziesmer, S. C., Witzig, T. E., & Ansell, S. M. (2009). Malignant B cells skew the balance of regulatory T cells and TH17 cells in B-cell non-Hodgkin's lymphoma. *Cancer research, 69*(13), 5522–5530. https://doi.org/10.1158/0008-5472.CAN-09-0266.

Yang, Z. Z., Grote, D. M., Ziesmer, S. C., Niki, T., Hirashima, M., Novak, A. J., Witzig, T. E., & Ansell, S. M. (2012). IL-12 upregulates TIM-3 expression and induces T cell exhaustion in patients with follicular B cell non-Hodgkin lymphoma. *Journal of Clinical Investigation, 122*(4), 1271–1282. https://doi.org/10.1172/JCI59806.

Yang, Z. Z., Grote, D. M., Xiu, B., Ziesmer, S. C., Price-Troska, T. L., Hodge, L. S., Yates, D. M., Novak, A. J., & Ansell, S. M. (2014). TGF-β upregulates CD70 expression and induces exhaustion of effector memory T cells in B-cell non-Hodgkin's lymphoma. *Leukemia*. Nature Publishing Group, *28*(October 2013), 1–13. https://doi.org/10.1038/leu.2014.84.

Yang, Z. Z., Liang, A. B., & Ansell, S. M. (2015). T-cell-mediated antitumor immunity in B-cell non-Hodgkin lymphoma: Activation, suppression and exhaustion. *Leukemia & lymphoma,* 1–16. https://doi.org/10.3109/10428194.2015.1011640.

Younes, A., Gopal, A. K., Smith, S. E., Ansell, S. M., Rosenblatt, J. D., Savage, K. J., Ramchandren, R., Bartlett, N. L., Cheson, B. D., De Vos, S., Forero-Torres, A., Moskowitz, C. H., Connors, J. M., Engert, A., Larsen, E. K., Kennedy, D. a., Sievers, E. L., & Chen, R. (2012). Results of a pivotal phase II study of brentuximab vedotin for patients with relapsed or refractory Hodgkin's lymphoma. *Journal of Clinical Oncology, 30*(18), 2183–2189. https://doi.org/10.1200/JCO.2011.38.0410.

Chapter 7
Combined Immunotherapy with Conventional Cancer Treatments

Yiyi Yan

Contents

Immunotherapy in Combination with Chemotherapy

For decades, cytotoxic chemotherapies have been the mainstay of treatment for many types of advanced malignancies until the recent revolutionary advances in cancer immunotherapy. However, considering that most patients will not show a durable response to immunotherapy, chemotherapy is still the most commonly used anticancer treatment, even in malignancies where immunotherapy is approved, especially in the setting of immune checkpoint inhibitor failure.

In patients who do not respond to immune checkpoint inhibitors, additional mechanisms of immunosuppression in the tumor microenvironment (within the tumors) and derangements in systemic immune competence (homeostasis) can drive chronic tumor-promoting inflammation, and therefore serve as potential barriers to treatment success (Gajewski 2006; Gajewski et al. 2006; Nevala et al. 2009). Overcoming these dysregulations is likely to improve PD-1 blockade efficacy. The immune system, both intratumoral and systemic, consists of many types of immune cells orchestrating the regulation of immune surveillance that leads to either tumor elimination or tumor growth and cancer metastasis. While some of those cells, such as CD8+ T cells and T helper 1 cells (Th1) (Haabeth et al. 2011), are responsible for anti-tumor activities, others play immunosuppressive roles promoting the tumor growth and invasion. Regulatory T cells (Treg), T-helper 2 cells (Th2) myeloid-derived suppressor cells (MDSC) (Bunt et al. 2007; Gabrilovich and Nagaraj 2009),

Y. Yan (✉)
Division of Medical Oncology, Mayo Clinic, Rochester, MN, USA

© Springer International Publishing AG 2018
H. Dong, S.N. Markovic (eds.), *The Basics of Cancer Immunotherapy*,
https://doi.org/10.1007/978-3-319-70622-1_7

and tumor-associated macrophages (TAM) are examples of immune cells that contribute to the suppressive immune environment favoring tumor progression. The disruption of the balance between the pro-tumorigenesis and anti-tumorigenic immune status can impact the outcome of the cancer immunotherapy.

Various types of chemotherapy drugs kill tumor cells through different mechanisms, such as inhibiting mitosis (a critical step in cell cycle progression) and DNA replication, as well as directly targeting cellular DNA or other key molecules that are critical for cancer cell division and survival. Interestingly, a delicate interplay between the effects of chemotherapy and one's immune system has been elucidated—the cell-killing induced by chemotherapies can modulate the immune system (both inside of the tumor and systemically), while the status of the immune system can impact the effectiveness of the chemotherapy drugs.

Anti-cancer cytotoxic chemotherapy has been regarded historically as detrimental to immunity because of its dose-limiting myelosuppression effects. However, recent discoveries have suggested that the anti-tumor effect of conventional cancer chemotherapy may result in part from its ability to disrupt immune suppressive pathways in addition to direct anti-tumor effects. For example, studies have shown that chemotherapy-induced lymphodepletion can counterintuitively augment anti-tumor immunity by potentiating tumor-specific T-cell responses (responsible for tumor killing) (Sampson et al. 2011; Williams et al. 2007). Possible mechanisms include depletion of Treg and other immunosuppressive cell populations (e.g., MDSCs, regulatory B cells), promotion of Th1/Th2 polarization, and enhanced proliferation of effector T-lymphocytes (Ghiringhelli et al. 2007; Alizadeh and Larmonier 2014). In addition, some chemotherapeutic agents promote anti-tumor immunity through induction of immunogenic cell death in tumors and depletion of immune-suppressor cells. Given the role of chemotherapy in overcoming the immune suppression that can result in resistance to immunotherapy, it has been hypothesized that immunotherapy in addition to chemotherapy may further activate the cytotoxic T cells with improved anti-tumor activities. This combination strategy has been investigated in multiple recent clinical trials.

For patients with non-small-cell lung cancer (NSCLC) clinical data for combinations of chemotherapy with anti-PD1 or anti-PD-L1 antibody (i.e., nivolumab and atezolizumab) have suggested that these regimens have promising anti-tumor activity and a manageable, non-overlapping toxicity profile (Rizvi et al. 2016; Camidge et al. 2015).

Pembrolizumab has recently received accelerated approval by the US Food and Drug Administration (FDA) for the treatment of NSCLC-adenocarcinomas in combination with carboplatin and pemetrexed in the first-line setting. In the clinical trial that led to this approval (Langer et al. 2016), a total of 123 chemo-naïve patients who were stratified by PD-L1 tumor cell expression ($< 1\%$ compared to $\geq 1\%$) were randomized to chemotherapy alone, or chemotherapy with pembrolizumab. Those who received chemotherapy alone could receive maintenance pemetrexed indefinitely, and those who received the combination of chemotherapy with pembrolizumab could receive maintenance pemetrexed indefinitely and pembrolizumab for up 24 months. The response rate was significantly higher for the chemotherapy-immunotherapy (CTIO) combination group (55%) than the chemotherapy alone group (29%). The progression-free survival was 13 months in the CTIO group versus 6 months in the chemotherapy alone group albeit with more toxicity (39% vs. 26% respectively). Response rates of patients treated with pembrolizumab and chemotherapy combination varied by PD-L1 tumor cell expression, such that the response rate of those with < 1% expression was 57%, those with ≥ 1% expression was 54%, those with 1–49% expression was 26%, and those with ≥ 50% expression was 80%. Accordingly, the expression of PD-L1 seems to enhance responses when a higher cutoff is used. This study supported CTIO as an alternative frontline therapeutic approach in non-squamous NSCLC patients who do not harbor targetable mutations and have < 50% tumor PD-L1 expression, since pembrolizumab is only indicated in those with ≥ 50% PD-L1 expression in this setting. In our practice, pembrolizumab monotherapy continues to be offered as the frontline therapy for NSCLC patients with tumor PD-L1 staining ≥ 50%, and targeted therapy should be offered for those with EGFR or ALK genetic alterations.

Multiple ongoing clinical trials are currently underway investigating the CTIO in other tumor types. For example, pembrolizumab in combination with different chemotherapy regimens are being tested in various types of advanced cancers in PembroPlus study (NCT02331251), pembrolizumab in combination with cisplatin or capecitabine or 5-Fluorouracil is being investigated in patients with gastric cancer in a KEYNOTE-062 study (NCT02494583).

Despite the effectiveness demonstrated in these trials, the efficacy and safety profile of CTIO combination therapies have significant room for further improvement. In order to develop the optimum therapeutic strategy, researchers need to further elucidate the mechanisms of chemo-induced regulation on immune responses augmented by immunotherapy, to develop the predictive and prognostic markers for patient selection and response assessment, and to define the sequence and timing of combination therapy. These are all areas of focus for recently emerging preclinical and clinical research activities over the last few years.

Chemotherapy can target proliferating cells besides cancer cells for killing, including lymphocytes. As we mentioned, these drugs can deplete immune suppressor cells, rendering an immune environment favoring anti-tumor activity. However, the impact of chemotherapy drugs on the function of tumor-reactive effector T cells is largely unknown. This is of particular importance because these types of T cells are mediators of the anti-tumor activity of immune checkpoint blockade. One of the research interests of our group is to identify the alterations that are caused by chemotherapy in this T cell population and the impacts of these alterations on the designs and outcomes of CTIO. We have recently discovered novel markers to identify human-reactive T cells and to monitor T cell response to anti-PD-1 therapy in melanoma patients. In one of our ongoing studies, we evaluated the impact of chemotherapy on these tumor-reactive T cells, taking advantage of samples from melanoma patients who failed initial pembrolizumab single therapy and received subsequent salvage CTIO combination (unpublished data). We found that a subpopulation of tumor-reactive T cells survived the chemotherapy treatment. More importantly, they are responsive to subsequent anti-PD-1 therapy with preserved antitumor activity. This unique subset of T cells plays a critical role in the success of CTIO and can be potentially developed as a biomarker to monitor the CTIO response.

The optimum sequence and timing of the CTIO therapy is still under investigation. In metastatic melanoma patients who have failed anti-PD1 therapy, chemotherapies are commonly offered as the next-line regimen. We have showed that approximately 26% of these patients demonstrated an objective response to subsequent chemotherapy (including carboplatin and paclitaxel) compared to a lower response rate in chemotherapy-treated historic controls (Flaherty et al. 2013), suggesting increased effectiveness of cytotoxic chemotherapy even after acquired resistance to PD-1 blockade compared to patients who have never received immunotherapy (Yan et al. 2016). Our preliminary results from melanoma animal models also demonstrated that chemotherapy after immunotherapy provides better tumor control compared to concurrent CTIO. In addition, the timing of the chemotherapy delivery also had a significant impact on the therapeutic effects. The sequence of CTIO has been controversial in both preclinical and clinical settings, and the optimum combination regimens are evolving. Further studies are warranted to address and evaluate these critical questions.

Immunotherapy in Combination with Targeted Therapy

The identification of tumor-specific driver mutations and deregulated signaling pathways has paved the way for the development of targeted therapy over the past few decades. These drugs have been widely incorporated into the management of various types of malignancies, including breast cancer (e.g., HER2 inhibitor), gastrointestinal cancers (e.g., EGFR inhibitors), gynecological cancers (e.g., PARP inhibitors), and melanoma (e.g., BRAF inhibitors), and have demonstrated effective clinical responses. Nevertheless, one of the major problems is the lack of response durability, underscoring the need to design alternative approaches to overcome the treatment resistance. Recent understanding of the immunoregulatory impact of these drugs has indicated that synergistic effects can be achieved through combining molecular targeted therapy with immune checkpoint inhibitors.

Preclinical models have demonstrated the importance of T-cell-dependent tumor killing in targeted therapies. For example, BRAF inhibitors can increase the CD8+ T cell infiltration into the tumors and decrease the immunosuppressive cytokines in metastatic melanoma patients, resulting in a favorable tumor microenvironment that correlates with tumor control (Wilmott et al. 2012). In a melanoma animal model, CD8+ T cells are required for the response to BRAF inhibitors (Knight et al. 2013; Cooper et al. 2014). In addition, its anti-tumor activity is enhanced when combined with PD-1 blockade. A currently ongoing phase 1/2 study is evaluating the efficacy and safety of pembrolizumab in combination with BRAF and MEK inhibitors (dabrafenib and trametinib) in patients with melanoma and other solid tumors (NCT02130466). Sorafenib, a multikinase inhibitor, can relieve the PD-1- and

Treg-mediated immunosuppression in a mouse model, promoting antitumor immunity (Chen et al. 2014). In an ongoing phase 1 trial (NCT03006926), pembrolizumab in combination with a tyrosine kinase inhibitor, lenvatinib, is being tested.

Olaparib is an oral poly (ADP-ribose) polymerase (PARP) inhibitor that has been used in ovarian cancers with BRCA1 and BRCA2 mutations. By inhibiting PARP, it can increase DNA damage frequencies, and therefore yield a greater mutational burden, leading to enhanced anti-tumor activity of immune cells. Interestingly, a recent animal study has demonstrated the immunoregulatory role of PARP inhibitors through increasing the peritoneal T-cell numbers (Huang et al. 2015). The combination of olaparib with durvalumab (a PD-L1 inhibitor) was recently investigated in a study that enrolled 26 women with gynecologic cancers. A disease control rate of 83% was reported with an acceptable safety profile, suggesting the therapeutic activity of this combination (Lee et al. 2017).

Antibodies targeting angiogenesis, such as bevacizumab (an anti-VEGF antibody) used in the treatment of colorectal and gynecologic cancers can also regulate the immune system through different mechanisms. For example, antiangiogenic agents can increase the T-cell infiltration with increased anti-tumor activity in an animal model (Manning et al. 2007). Bevacizumab can decrease Treg and MDSC populations in colorectal cancer (Terme et al. 2013). In addition, the resultant hypoxic conditions can upregulate PD-L1 expression. These data suggest that angiogenesis inhibition in combination with immune checkpoint inhibitors can enhance the anti-tumor response. A recent clinical trial using a combination of bevacizumab and ipilimumab (anti-CTLA4 antibody) has demonstrated a clinical benefit in melanoma patients (Hodi et al. 2014). The combination of bevacizumab with pembrolizumab is under current investigation in patients with ovarian cancer (NCT02853318) and patients with brain metastases from solid tumors (NCT02681549).

With the growing lists of targeted drugs and immune checkpoint inhibitors, immunomodulatory mechanisms of this combination need to be further elucidated in order to develop more efficacious therapies.

Immunotherapy in Combination with Radiation Therapy

Radiation therapy (RT) is used as a definitive or palliative treatment modality in different types of malignancies. In addition to controlling tumor growth and promoting immunogenic cell death, RT regulates the immune response both systemically and within the tumor microenvironment. For example, the abscopal effect, a clinical phenomenon referring to the distant systemic tumor response in the unirradiated tumors after localized radiation delivery to tumors, is a result of RT-induced immune modulations. In the era of novel cancer immunotherapy, RT has gained attention from researchers for the potential synergistic response in combination with immune checkpoint inhibitors.

Although historically considered to be immunosuppressive due to myelosuppression, RT has been shown to modulate immune responses through multiple mechanisms (Barker et al. 2015). RT can increase the recruitment of cytotoxic T cells to the tumor microenvironment through the release of chemokines (Matsumura et al. 2008); augment the T-cell tumor recognition by upregulating the key cell surface molecules (including antigen presentation machinery) (Reits et al. 2006; Kim et al., 2006); enhance the priming of the T cells for activation (Gupta et al. 2012; Gameiro et al. 2014); upregulate PD-L1 expression in the tumor microenvironment (Deng et al. 2014); and alter the immunosuppressive tumor microenvironment with resultant accessibility for T-cell infiltration (Klug et al. 2013). In a mouse breast cancer model, RT in combination with anti-CTLA4 antibody delayed tumor growth, decreased metastasis, and improved survival (Demaria et al. 2005). In NSCLC mouse models, RT in combination with an anti-PD1 agent induced significant and long-lasting tumor response (Herter-Sprie et al. 2016).

The combination of RT with immune checkpoint inhibitors has recently been investigated, although data supporting its routine clinical application remain limited. In a study conducted in melanoma patients, the combination of RT and ipilimumab did not increase the risk of immune-related adverse events. However, no survival benefit was observed (Barker et al. 2013). In the secondary analysis of phase 1 KEYNOTE-001 study (Shaverdian et al. 2017), NSCLC patients who received pembrolizumab after RT had better survival than those who had not undergone RT prior to pembrolizumab, suggesting the potential activity of the RT-immunotherapy combination. Durvalumab, an anti-PDL1 antibody, was recently examined in the phase 3 randomized PACIFIC trial in stage III NSCLC patients who received definitive chemoradiation (NCT02125461) (Antonia et al. 2017). A total of 713 patients underwent randomization to either durvalumab consolidation or placebo in a 2:1 ratio and patients were not selected for their PD-L1 expression. Durvalumab significantly improved the median progression survival compared to placebo (16.8 months vs. 5.6 months). The 12-month progression survival rate was 55.9% in the durvalumab versus 35.5% in the placebo group. Despite the encouraging results from this study, further investigation is warranted to elucidate the mechanism of the interaction between RT, chemo-, and immunotherapy, and to develop optimized combination strategies. Multiple clinical trials are currently ongoing to evaluate the combination of RT and immunotherapy, including NCT02830594 in metastatic GI malignancies and NCT02730130 for metastatic breast cancer.

Conclusion

Current pre-clinical and clinical research in cancer immunotherapy are focused on modulating host immune response through two main approaches—increasing the cancer-killing ability of the immune system (e.g., boosting the T-cell function via checkpoint inhibitors) and suppressing the tumor-promoting immune process. The recent unprecedented success of immune checkpoint inhibitors in cancer treatment has rapidly reinvigorated the field of oncology and cancer research. Given the fact that they do not provide clinical benefit in the majority of cancer patients, it is crucial to design efficacious synergic therapeutic approaches with increased response. Chemotherapy, radiation therapy, and targeted therapy have been shown to modulate the host immune system, making it more favorable for T-cell anti-tumor activity enhanced by immune checkpoint inhibitor. Although these combinations have shown some promising results in clinical studies, further research is needed to elucidate the exact immune-regulatory mechanisms and the treatment strategies, such as regimen, dose, and schedule, of the combination therapy.

References

Alizadeh, D., & Larmonier, N. (2014). Chemotherapeutic targeting of cancer-induced immunosuppressive cells. *Cancer Research, 74*, 2663–2668.

Antonia, S. J., Villegas, A., Daniel, D., Vicente, D., Murakami, S., Hui, R., Yokoi, T., Chiappori, A., Lee, K. H., De Wit, M., Cho, B. C., Bourhaba, M., Quantin, X., Tokito, T., Mekhail, T., Planchard, D., Kim, Y. C., Karapetis, C. S., Hiret, S., Ostoros, G., Kubota, K., Gray, J. E., Paz-Ares, L., De Castro Carpeno, J., Wadsworth, C., Melillo, G., Jiang, H., Huang, Y., Dennis, P. A., Ozguroglu, M., & Investigators, P. (2017). Durvalumab after chemoradiotherapy in stage III non-small-cell lung cancer. The *New England Journal of Medicine, 377*, 1919–1929.

Barker, C. A., Postow, M. A., Khan, S. A., Beal, K., Parhar, P. K., Yamada, Y., Lee, N. Y., & Wolchok, J. D. (2013). Concurrent radiotherapy and ipilimumab immunotherapy for patients with melanoma. *Cancer Immunology Research, 1*, 92–98.

Barker, H. E., Paget, J. T., Khan, A. A., & Harrington, K. J. (2015). The tumour microenvironment after radiotherapy: Mechanisms of resistance and recurrence. *Nature Reviews. Cancer, 15*, 409–425.

Bunt, S. K., Yang, L., Sinha, P., Clements, V. K., Leips, J., & Ostrand-Rosenberg, S. (2007). Reduced inflammation in the tumor microenvironment delays the accumulation of myeloid-derived suppressor cells and limits tumor progression. *Cancer Research, 67*, 10019–10026.

Camidge, R., Liu, S. V., Powderly, J., Ready, N., Hodi, S., Gettinger, S. N., Giaccone, G., Liu, B., Wallin, J., Funke, R., Waterkamp, D., & Heist, R. (2015). Atezolizumab (MPDL3280A) combined with platinum-based chemotherapy in Non-Small Cell Lung Cancer (NSCLC): A Phase Ib Safety and Efficacy Update. *Journal of Thoracic Oncology, 10*, S176–S177.

Chen, M. L., Yan, B. S., Lu, W. C., Chen, M. H., Yu, S. L., Yang, P. C., & Cheng, A. L. (2014). Sorafenib relieves cell-intrinsic and cell-extrinsic inhibitions of effector T cells in tumor microenvironment to augment anti-tumor immunity. *International Journal of Cancer, 134*, 319–331.

Cooper, Z. A., Juneja, V. R., Sage, P. T., Frederick, D. T., Piris, A., Mitra, D., Lo, J. A., Hodi, F. S., Freeman, G. J., Bosenberg, M. W., Mcmahon, M., Flaherty, K. T., Fisher, D. E., Sharpe, A. H., & Wargo, J. A. (2014). Response to BRAF inhibition in melanoma is enhanced when combined with immune checkpoint blockade. *Cancer Immunology Research, 2*, 643–654.

Demaria, S., Kawashima, N., Yang, A. M., Devitt, M. L., Babb, J. S., Allison, J. P., & Formenti, S. C. (2005). Immune-mediated inhibition of metastases after treatment with local radiation and CTLA-4 blockade in a mouse model of breast cancer. *Clinical Cancer Research, 11*, 728–734.

Deng, L., Liang, H., Burnette, B., Beckett, M., Darga, T., Weichselbaum, R. R., & Fu, Y. X. (2014). Irradiation and anti-PD-L1 treatment synergistically promote anti-tumor immunity in mice. *The Journal of Clinical Investigation, 124*, 687–695.

Flaherty, K. T., Lee, S. J., Zhao, F., Schuchter, L. M., Flaherty, L., Kefford, R., Atkins, M. B., Leming, P., & Kirkwood, J. M. (2013). Phase III trial of carboplatin and paclitaxel with or without sorafenib in metastatic melanoma. *Journal of Clinical Oncology, 31*, 373–379.

Gabrilovich, D. I., & Nagaraj, S. (2009). Myeloid-derived suppressor cells as regulators of the immune system. *Nature Reviews. Immunology, 9*, 162–174.

Gajewski, T. F. (2006). Identifying and overcoming immune resistance mechanisms in the melanoma tumor microenvironment. *Clinical Cancer Research, 12*, 2326s–2330s.

Gajewski, T. F., Meng, Y., Blank, C., Brown, I., Kacha, A., Kline, J., & Harlin, H. (2006). Immune resistance orchestrated by the tumor microenvironment. *Immunological Reviews, 213*, 131–145.

Gameiro, S. R., Ardiani, A., Kwilas, A., & Hodge, J. W. (2014). Radiation-induced survival responses promote immunogenic modulation to enhance immunotherapy in combinatorial regimens. *Oncoimmunology, 3*, e28643.

Ghiringhelli, F., Menard, C., Puig, P. E., Ladoire, S., Roux, S., Martin, F., Solary, E., Le Cesne, A., Zitvogel, L., & Chauffert, B. (2007). Metronomic cyclophosphamide regimen selectively depletes CD4+CD25+ regulatory T cells and restores T and NK effector functions in end stage cancer patients. *Cancer Immunology, Immunotherapy, 56*, 641–648.

Gupta, A., Probst, H. C., Vuong, V., Landshammer, A., Muth, S., Yagita, H., Schwendener, R., Pruschy, M., Knuth, A., & Van Den Broek, M. (2012). Radiotherapy promotes tumor-specific effector CD8+ T cells via dendritic cell activation. *Journal of Immunology, 189*, 558–566.

Haabeth, O. A., Lorvik, K. B., Hammarstrom, C., Donaldson, I. M., Haraldsen, G., Bogen, B., & Corthay, A. (2011). Inflammation driven by tumour-specific Th1 cells protects against B-cell cancer. *Nature Communications, 2*, 240.

Herter-Sprie, G. S., Koyama, S., Korideck, H., Hai, J., Deng, J., Li, Y. Y., Buczkowski, K. A., Grant, A. K., Ullas, S., Rhee, K., Cavanaugh, J. D., Neupane, N. P., Christensen, C. L., Herter, J. M., Makrigiorgos, G. M., Hodi, F. S., Freeman, G. J., Dranoff, G., Hammerman, P. S., Kimmelman, A. C., & Wong, K. K. (2016). Synergy of radiotherapy and PD-1 blockade in Kras-mutant lung cancer. *JCI Insight, 1*, e87415.

Hodi, F. S., Lawrence, D., Lezcano, C., Wu, X., Zhou, J., Sasada, T., Zeng, W., Giobbie-Hurder, A., Atkins, M. B., Ibrahim, N., Friedlander, P., Flaherty, K. T., Murphy, G. F., Rodig, S., Velazquez, E. F., Mihm, M. C., Jr., Russell, S., Dipiro, P. J., Yap, J. T., Ramaiya, N., Van Den Abbeele, A. D., Gargano, M., & Mcdermott, D. (2014). Bevacizumab plus ipilimumab in patients with metastatic melanoma. *Cancer Immunology Research, 2*, 632–642.

Huang, J., Wang, L., Cong, Z., Amoozgar, Z., Kiner, E., Xing, D., Orsulic, S., Matulonis, U., & Goldberg, M. S. (2015). The PARP1 inhibitor BMN 673 exhibits immunoregulatory effects in a Brca1(−/−) murine model of ovarian cancer. *Biochemical and Biophysical Research Communications, 463*, 551–556.

Kim, J. Y., Son, Y. O., Park, S. W., Bae, J. H., Chung, J. S., Kim, H. H., Chung, B. S., Kim, S. H., & Kang, C. D. (2006). Increase of NKG2D ligands and sensitivity to NK cell-mediated cytotoxicity of tumor cells by heat shock and ionizing radiation. *Experimental & Molecular Medicine, 38*, 474–484.

Klug, F., Prakash, H., Huber, P. E., Seibel, T., Bender, N., Halama, N., Pfirschke, C., Voss, R. H., Timke, C., Umansky, L., Klapproth, K., Schakel, K., Garbi, N., Jager, D., Weitz, J., Schmitz-Winnenthal, H., Hammerling, G. J., & Beckhove, P. (2013). Low-dose irradiation programs macrophage differentiation to an iNOS(+)/M1 phenotype that orchestrates effective T cell immunotherapy. *Cancer Cell, 24*, 589–602.

Knight, D. A., Ngiow, S. F., Li, M., Parmenter, T., Mok, S., Cass, A., Haynes, N. M., Kinross, K., Yagita, H., Koya, R. C., Graeber, T. G., Ribas, A., Mcarthur, G. A., & Smyth, M. J. (2013). Host immunity contributes to the anti-melanoma activity of BRAF inhibitors. *The Journal of Clinical Investigation, 123*, 1371–1381.

Langer, C. J., Gadgeel, S. M., Borghaei, H., Papadimitrakopoulou, V. A., Patnaik, A., Powell, S. F., Gentzler, R. D., Martins, R. G., Stevenson, J. P., Jalal, S. I., Panwalkar, A., Yang, J. C., Gubens, M., Sequist, L. V., Awad, M. M., Fiore, J., Ge, Y., Raftopoulos, H., Gandhi, L., & Investigators, K. (2016). Carboplatin and pemetrexed with or without pembrolizumab for advanced, non-squamous non-small-cell lung cancer: A randomised, phase 2 cohort of the open-label KEYNOTE-021 study. *The Lancet Oncology, 17*, 1497–1508.

Lee, J. M., Cimino-Mathews, A., Peer, C. J., Zimmer, A., Lipkowitz, S., Annunziata, C. M., Cao, L., Harrell, M. I., Swisher, E., Houston, N., Botesteanu, D. A., Taube, J. M., Thompson, E.,

Ogurtsova, A., Xu, H. Y., Nguyen, J., Ho, T. W., Figg, W. D., & Kohn, E. C. (2017). Safety and clinical activity of the programmed death-ligand 1 inhibitor durvalumab in combination with Poly (ADP-Ribose) polymerase inhibitor olaparib or vascular endothelial growth factor receptor 1-3 inhibitor cediranib in women's cancers: A dose-escalation, phase I study. *Journal of Clinical Oncology, 35*, 2193–2202.

Manning, E. A., Ullman, J. G., Leatherman, J. M., Asquith, J. M., Hansen, T. R., Armstrong, T. D., Hicklin, D. J., Jaffee, E. M., & Emens, L. A. (2007). A vascular endothelial growth factor receptor-2 inhibitor enhances anti-tumor immunity through an immune-based mechanism. *Clinical Cancer Research, 13*, 3951–3959.

Matsumura, S., Wang, B., Kawashima, N., Braunstein, S., Badura, M., Cameron, T. O., Babb, J. S., Schneider, R. J., Formenti, S. C., Dustin, M. L., & Demaria, S. (2008). Radiation-induced CXCL16 release by breast cancer cells attracts effector T cells. *Journal of Immunology, 181*, 3099–3107.

Nevala, W. K., Vachon, C. M., Leontovich, A. A., Scott, C. G., Thompson, M. A., Markovic, S. N., & Melanoma Study Group Of The Mayo Clinic Cancer, C. (2009). Evidence of systemic Th2-driven chronic inflammation in patients with metastatic melanoma. *Clinical Cancer Research, 15*, 1931–1939.

Reits, E. A., Hodge, J. W., Herberts, C. A., Groothuis, T. A., Chakraborty, M., Wansley, E. K., Camphausen, K., Luiten, R. M., De Ru, A. H., Neijssen, J., Griekspoor, A., Mesman, E., Verreck, F. A., Spits, H., Schlom, J., Van veelen, P., & Neefjes, J. J. (2006). Radiation modulates the peptide repertoire, enhances MHC class I expression, and induces successful anti-tumor immunotherapy. *The Journal of Experimental Medicine, 203*, 1259–1271.

Ribas, A., Hamid, O., Daud, A., Hodi, F. S., Wolchok, J. D., Kefford, R., Joshua, A. M., Patnaik, A., Hwu, W. J., Weber, J. S., Gangadhar, T. C., Hersey, P., Dronca, R., Joseph, R. W., Zarour, H., Chmielowski, B., Lawrence, D. P., Algazi, A., Rizvi, N. A., Hoffner, B., Mateus, C., Gergich, K., Lindia, J. A., Giannotti, M., Li, X. N., Ebbinghaus, S., Kang, S. P., & Robert, C. (2016). Association of pembrolizumab with tumor response and survival among patients with advanced melanoma. *JAMA, 315*, 1600–1609.

Rizvi, N. A., Hellmann, M. D., Brahmer, J. R., Juergens, R. A., Borghaei, H., Gettinger, S., Chow, L. Q., Gerber, D. E., Laurie, S. A., Goldman, J. W., Shepherd, F. A., Chen, A. C., Shen, Y., Nathan, F. E., Harbison, C. T., & Antonia, S. (2016). Nivolumab in combination with platinum-based doublet chemotherapy for first-line treatment of advanced non-small-cell lung cancer. *Journal of Clinical Oncology, 34*, 2969–2979.

Sampson, J. H., Aldape, K. D., Archer, G. E., Coan, A., Desjardins, A., Friedman, A. H., Friedman, H. S., Gilbert, M. R., Herndon, J. E., Mclendon, R. E., Mitchell, D. A., Reardon, D. A., Sawaya, R., Schmittling, R., Shi, W., Vredenburgh, J. J., Bigner, D. D., & Heimberger, A. B. (2011). Greater chemotherapy-induced lymphopenia enhances tumor-specific immune responses that eliminate EGFRvIII-expressing tumor cells in patients with glioblastoma. *Neuro-Oncology, 13*, 324–333.

Shaverdian, N., Lisberg, A. E., Bornazyan, K., Veruttipong, D., Goldman, J. W., Formenti, S. C., Garon, E. B., & Lee, P. (2017). Previous radiotherapy and the clinical activity and toxicity of pembrolizumab in the treatment of non-small-cell lung cancer: A secondary analysis of the KEYNOTE-001 phase 1 trial. *The Lancet Oncology, 18*, 895–903.

Terme, M., Pernot, S., Marcheteau, E., Sandoval, F., Benhamouda, N., Colussi, O., Dubreuil, O., Carpentier, A. F., Tartour, E., & Taieb, J. (2013). VEGFA-VEGFR pathway blockade inhibits tumor-induced regulatory T-cell proliferation in colorectal cancer. *Cancer Research, 73*, 539–549.

Williams, K. M., Hakim, F. T., & Gress, R. E. (2007). T cell immune reconstitution following lymphodepletion. *Seminars in Immunology, 19*, 318–330.

Wilmott, J. S., Long, G. V., Howle, J. R., Haydu, L. E., Sharma, R. N., Thompson, J. F., Kefford, R. F., Hersey, P., & Scolyer, R. A. (2012). Selective BRAF inhibitors induce marked T-cell infiltration into human metastatic melanoma. *Clinical Cancer Research, 18*, 1386–1394.

Yan, Y., Failing, J., Leontovich, A. A., Block, M. S., Mcwilliams, R. R., Kottschade, L. A., Dronca, R. S., & Markovic, S. (2016). The Mayo Clinic experience in patients with metastatic melanoma who have failed previous pembrolizumab treatment. *ASCO Meeting Abstracts, 34*, e21014.

Chapter 8
Immunotherapy for Other Malignancies

Yiyi Yan

Contents

Breast Cancer

In the USA, about one in eight females will be diagnosed with invasive breast cancer during their lifetime. It is the leading cancer diagnosis (estimated 262,710 cases) and second leading cause of cancer death (estimated 40,610 cases) for females in 2017 (cancer.org). While significant advances have been made in the treatment of estrogen receptor (ER)-positive and/or HER2-positive breast cancer over the past few decades, no novel agents have been approved for the treatment of triple negative breast cancer [(TNBC) ER−/PR−/HER2-]. The management of TNBC, the most aggressive subtype, is still limited to traditional cytotoxic chemotherapy, and the outcomes remain inferior to other subtypes. Although breast cancer as a whole is considered to be less immunogenic compared to other cancers such as melanoma, TNBC and HER2+ breast cancers appear to be more immunogenic. These breast cancer subtypes exhibit higher levels of tumor-infiltrating lymphocytes (TILs), including T cells and B cells, in the tumor microenvironment. The levels of TILs have been shown to correlate

Y. Yan (✉)
Division of Medical Oncology, Mayo Clinic, Rochester, MN, USA

© Springer International Publishing AG 2018
H. Dong, S.N. Markovic (eds.), *The Basics of Cancer Immunotherapy*,
https://doi.org/10.1007/978-3-319-70622-1_8

with disease prognosis and responses to both neoadjuvant and adjuvant chemotherapy (Salgado et al. 2015; Denkert et al. 2010; Ali et al. 2014).

PD-L1 expression is highly heterogeneous across different breast cancer subtypes, and it is associated with clinicopathological features such as lymphocyte infiltration, aggressive subtypes, and poor prognosis; however, inconsistent results have been shown depending on the test methods and platforms (Sabatier et al. 2015; Ali et al. 2015). These findings have led to further clinical efforts to explore the role of immunotherapies for patients with metastatic breast cancers.

PD-1 and PD-L1 inhibitors (pembrolizumab and atezolizumab or avelumab, respectively) have been investigated in multiple clinical trials for their safety and anti-tumor activities. Pembrolizumab was studied in KEYNOTE-012 (ClinicalTrials. gov identifier: NCT01848834), a non-randomized phase 1b trial on patients with TNBC (Nanda et al. 2016). Patients with PD-L expression of $\geq$ 1% of tumor cells by immunohistochemistry in tumor stroma (58.6% of screened patients using archived tissues) received pembrolizumab at 10 mg/kg every 2 weeks. All patients received at least one line of previous therapy before being enrolled into the study. Pembrolizumab was well tolerated and provided an overall response rate (ORR) of 18.5% with a disease control rate of 25.9% and a median time to response of 17.9 weeks. The 6-month progression-free survival (PFS) was 24.4% and median overall survival (OS) was > 11 months. This study established the clinical safety profile and clinical activity, and a phase 2 study for single-agent pembrolizumab in advanced TNBC patients is currently ongoing (NCT02447003). In this study, cohort A consisted of previously treated metastatic TNBC regardless of tumor PD-L1 expression. Of 170 patients, 61.8% were PD-L1 positive, 37.6% were PD-L1 negative, and 0.6% were PD-L1 unknown. After a median follow-up of 10.9 months, the ORR was 4.7% and the disease control rate was 7.6%. Interestingly, there was no difference in response rate for PD-L1-positive versus PD-L1-negative cohorts. All patients with complete or partial responses were still alive at the time of data analysis. The 6-month PFS and OS rates were 12% and 69%, respectively. Pembrolizumab was also studied in ER+/HER2- breast cancer patients with positive PD-L1 expression in KEYNOTE-028 (NCT02054806). An overall response rate of 12% with a well-tolerated safety profile was reported.

In addition, pembrolizumab has been evaluated in the neoadjuvant setting in the I-SPY 2 clinical trial, a phase 2 adaptively randomized, controlled, multicenter trial evaluating novel neoadjuvant therapies in women with newly diagnosed, locally advanced breast cancers. The primary endpoint of this study is pathologic complete response (defined as no residual invasive cancer in the breast or lymph nodes). This study included patients of all breast cancer subtypes at high risk of relapse (based on upfront tumor profiling). Patients were randomized to standard neoadjuvant chemotherapy with or without pembrolizumab. In patients with TNBC, the addition of pembrolizumab tripled the estimated pathologic complete response rate from 20% to 60%. Interestingly, in patients with ER-positive, HER2-negative breast cancer (traditionally considered less immunogenic), addition of pembrolizumab led to an absolute increase in the estimated pathologic complete response rate of 21%.

Atezolizumab was also evaluated in heavily treated metastatic TNBC patients in a phase 1 study (NCT01375842) (Emens et al. 2015). When given at a 3-weekly schedule, atezolizumab had an acceptable toxicity profile providing an ORR of 24% with a 24-week PFS rate of 33% in patients with PD-L1 positive tumors. Avelumab, a PD-L1 inhibitor, was studied in the phase 1b JAVELIN trial (NCT01772004) (Dirix et al. 2016). Previously treated metastatic cancer patients regardless of ER/PR/HER2 and PD-L status were enrolled. A lower ORR was observed (8.8%; 95% confidence interval (CI): 2.9–9.3) in 57 TNBC patients compared to trials with pembrolizumab and atezolizumab. In patients with non-TNBC, only two out of 72 patients had an objective response.

These studies provided clinical evidence supporting the anti-tumor activities of immune checkpoint inhibitors in advanced breast cancer, especially in metastatic TNBC. However, biomarker testing and selection for optimization of treatment response needs further investigation.

To further improve the clinical outcomes, additional treatment strategies are currently being investigated. Clinical trials are designed to evaluate the safety and efficacy using immunotherapy in combination with chemotherapy/biological agents (e.g., PembroPlus (NCT02331251), KEYNOTE-162 (NCT02657889)), or in early stages and the preoperative setting (NCT02957968).

Gastrointestinal Cancer

Gastrointestinal (GI) cancer remains the most common tumor worldwide. Despite multiple screening methods and treatment modalities, the incidence and mortality continue to increase with these tumors. The advances in modern immunotherapies with checkpoint inhibitors provide a unique opportunity to improve the outcomes in patients with advanced GI cancers. The issue of using biomarkers (e.g., PD-L1 expression) to predict benefits from immunotherapy is in evolution. Herein, we will briefly review the recent clinical data of immune checkpoint inhibitors in the management of esophageal, gastric (including gastro-esophageal junction (GEJ)), colorectal, hepatobiliary, and pancreatic cancer.

Esophageal Cancer

Esophageal cancer is the sixth leading cause of cancer-related death in the world (Ferlay et al. 2015), and is one of the less studied malignancies. A multidisciplinary approach (surgery and radiation) and chemotherapy have been the standard-of-care for decades. Fortunately, the development of cancer immunotherapies is changing the landscape of its management. Genetic and immunological studies had revealed a few interesting features of esophageal cancers that supported the potential utilization of immunotherapy checkpoint. It has been reported that tumors from esophageal cancers carry a high somatic mutation rate, which is considered to be associated with better clinical responses to anti-PD-1 therapy (Segal et al. 2008; Lawrence et al. 2013; Rizvi et al. 2015). In addition, overexpression of PD-1 ligands was found in over 40% of esophageal cancer tumor samples (Ohigashi et al. 2005).

Pembrolizumab, an anti-PD-1 monoclonal antibody, has been studied in multiple clinical trials for patients with advanced esophageal cancer with PD-L1 expression. In the abovementioned KEYNOTE-012 (NCT01848834) (Doi et al. 2015), a phase 1b study enrolling patients with > 1% of PD-L1 expression in tumors, 23 patients with pretreated esophageal cancer were given pembrolizumab. An ORR of 30.4% (40.0% for adenocarcinoma, 29.4% for squamous cell) and stable disease rate (SD) of 13% was observed, with 6-month PFS of 30.4% and 12-month PFS of 21.7%, indicating a meaningful activity of pembrolizumab in PD-L1+ advanced esophageal cancer. Nivolumab is another PD-1 inhibitor that has been investigated in patients with advanced esophageal cancer. In a single-arm multicenter phase 2 study (Kudo et al. 2017), 65 patients (squamous, adenosquamous, or adenocarcinoma histology) who failed previous chemotherapy were enrolled and received nivolumab once every 2 weeks. Importantly, patients were not selected according to their tumor PD-L1 expression levels. Objective response was seen in 17% (95% CI: 10–28) of patients, with a manageable toxicity profile. These results demonstrated that PD-1 blockade is a potential treatment in patients with esophageal cancer who failed previous chemotherapy; however, the role of PD-L1 testing in patient selection needs further investigation. There are multiple ongoing large phase 3 trials validating the role of anti-PD-1 antibodies in the treatment of advanced recurrent esophageal cancer, including nivolumab (NCT02569242) and pembrolizumab (NCT02564263).

The clinical response and durability of PD-1 inhibitors alone remain limited. In order to improve the outcomes, combination strategies are currently being investigated in patients with esophageal cancer, including combinations of cancer immunotherapies, immunotherapy with radiation, and immunotherapy with chemotherapies. PD-1 blockade in combination with anti-CTLA-4 blockade (ipilimumab) has been shown to have a high response rate in patients with metastatic melanoma (ref). This result has led to multiple trials testing this combination in other solid tumors, including esophageal cancer (UMIN00002148). Radiation therapy (RT) is the foundation of esophageal cancer treatment, either in the perioperative or palliative setting. The immunoregulatory effects of RT led to clinical studies investigating its combination with immune checkpoint inhibitors. Trials of pembrolizumab in combination with RT are currently underway in metastatic esophageal patients (NCT02642809; NCT02830594). Patients with advanced esophageal cancer were also included in the abovementioned PembroPlus trial, combining pembrolizumab with chemotherapies. The results of these ongoing clinical studies will further change the paradigm of esophageal cancer management.

Gastric and Gastroesophageal Junction Cancer

PD-L1 overexpression has been detected in gastric patients, especially in Epstein-Barr virus (EBV)-positive and microsatellite instable subtypes (Derks et al. 2016), and is associated with large tumors and lymph node metastases with a poor prognosis (Zhang et al. 2016; Liu et al. 2016). Patients with recurrent or metastatic gastric or gastroesophageal junction (GEJ) adenocarcinoma with $\geq$ 1% PD-L1 expression were enrolled into the KEYNOTE-012 trial and treated with pembrolizumab (Muro et al. 2016). Among 39 enrolled patients, 36 were evaluable for disease response. The ORR was 22% (95% CI: 10–39) by central review, and median response duration was 24 weeks (range 8+ to 33+). In the phase 2 KEYNOTE-059 trial (NCT02335411) (Charles S. Fuchs et al. 2017), 259 patients with advanced gastric or GEJ cancer who had progressed on at least two prior chemotherapy regimens were treated with pembrolizumab. A total of 143 these patients had PD-L1+ tumors ($\geq$ 1%). The ORR was 13.3% in the PD-L1 positive cohort with a complete response rate of 1.4% and a partial response rate of 11.9%. The US Food and Drug Administration (FDA) recently approved keytruday for the treatment of recurrent locally advanced or metastatic gastric or GEJ cancer with positive PD-L1 expression.

Nivolumab is another PD-1 blockade that has been shown to be effective in gastric and GEJ cancers with improved outcomes. In a phase 3 trial, a total of 493 patients (Asian population, non-selective for PD-L1 expression) who failed previous chemotherapies were enrolled and received either nivolumab or placebo (Kang et al. 2017). The preliminary results showed a median OS of 5.3 months with nivolumab versus 4.14 months with placebo. OS rates at 6 and 12 months were 46.4% versus 34.7% and 26.6% versus 10.9%, respectively. The ORR was 11.2% with nivolumab versus 0% with placebo. The clinical benefit of nivolumab in a western population was recently evaluated in the CheckMate 032 study, enrolling 160 previously treated patients with esophageal, gastric, or GEJ cancer (24% with PD-L1+ tumors). Among 59 patients who received nivolumab (3 mg/kg), ORR was 12% (19% in PD-L1+ population) with a median duration of response of 7.1 months.

Clinical trials investigating immune checkpoint inhibitors in combination with other therapies are also being performed. Pembrolizumab combined with chemotherapy (cisplatin plus 5-fluorouracil) versus pembrolizumab alone is being evaluated in patients with recurrent or metastatic gastric or GEJ cancer (NCT01928394). Nivolumab in combination with ipilimumab (anti-CTLA-4 antibody) is currently being tested for its safety and efficacy in clinical trial NCT01928394 for patients with gastric cancer.

Hepatobiliary Cancer

Hepatocellular carcinoma (HCC) is the most common primary liver malignancy. It usually occurs in the setting of chronic liver disease, such as viral hepatitis and cirrhosis, and is aggressive with a poor overall prognosis. Treatment options include curative surgical resection, transplantation, and liver-directed treatment. Systemic therapies, such as chemotherapy, molecular targeting therapy, and hormone therapy, are of very limited benefit. The immunoregulatory pathways have been studied in HCC tumors. It has been reported that PD-L1 is highly expressed in HCC tumor cells and surrounding immune cells and the overexpression of PD-L1 is correlated with aggressive clinical features and worse survival (Wang et al. 2011; Gao et al. 2009), suggesting a potential therapeutic role of PD-1 blockade in HCC by restoring anti-tumor immunity .

In CheckMate 040, a phase 1/2 trial, nivolumab was evaluated in advanced HCC patients (with or without hepatitis C or B (HCV or HBV) infection) who had progressed on or were intolerant of sorafenib (El-Khoueiry et al. 2017). This trial included a dose-escalation cohort (48 patients) and an expansion cohort (214 patients). In the dose-escalation phase, the maximum tolerated dose was not reached (at 0.1–10 mg/kg every 2 weeks), and the tolerability and safety profile were acceptable. In the dose-expansion phase, patients were treated with nivolumab at 3 mg/kg, and the reported ORR was 20% (95% CI: 15–26), and the 9 months OS was 74% with a median duration of response (DOR) of 9.9 months. These durable benefits were observed both in sorafenib-naïve and sorafenib-experienced patients with ORR of 23% and 16%, respectively (Crocenzi et al. 2017). Results from this study strongly support future investigations to establish the role of immune checkpoint inhibitors in the treatment of HCC. Nivolumab gained FDA approval for the treatment of HCC in patients previously treated with sorafenib. In an ongoing phase 3 study (KEYNOTE-240, NCT02702401), pembrolizumab versus best supportive care is being tested in patients with advanced HCC who have received previous systemic treatment.

Combination approaches also have been explored in HCC treatment aiming to improve the overall outcomes. For example, nivolumab in combination with ipilimumab is being evaluated in CheckMate 040 (NCT 01658878), and pembrolizumab in combination with a tyrosine kinase inhibitor, lenvatinib, is being tested in a phase 1 trial (NCT03006926).

Cholangiocarcinoma is a cancer arising from the epithelial cells of the bile ducts. Patients usually present with advanced disease and have a high mortality rate. Systemic chemotherapy is the standard-of-care for patients with good performance status who have non-resectable diseases, although the survival benefit is minimal. Anti-PD-1 antibodies have recently been investigated for patients with cholangiocarcinoma since PD-L1 expression was found to be upregulated and associated with a poor prognosis (Gani et al. 2016). In KEYNOTE-028 (Bang et al. 2015), 24 patients with PD-L1+ biliary tract cancer received pembrolizumab. An ORR of 17% was reported.

Pancreatic Cancer

Pancreatic cancer remains an aggressive and lethal disease despite recent advances in the understanding of the biological mechanisms underlying its pathogenesis. Although surgical resection offers an opportunity for cure, the majority of the patients (> 80%) present with unresectable locally advanced or metastatic disease at the time of diagnosis. The immunosuppressive tumor microenvironment of pancreatic cancer is attributed to the extremely poor treatment response and is one of the obstacles in therapy development.

Immune checkpoint inhibitors have been tested in multiple clinical trials for advanced pancreatic adenocarcinoma. In a phase 2 study (Royal et al. 2010), 27 patients were treated with ipilimumab and no responders were observed. In another phase 1 trial (Brahmer et al. 2012), 0 out of 14 pancreatic cancer patients treated with MDX1105–11 (PD-L1inhibitor) experienced an objective response. A recent early-phase study (NCT01693562) investigated the safety and efficacy of durvalumab (PD-L1 blockade) in multiple solid tumors, including 29 pancreatic cancer patients (Segal et al. 2014). An ORR of 7% and 12-week disease control rate (DCR) of 21% was observed. Phase 2 studies are currently ongoing to further test the efficacy of durvalumab (NCT02558894). Although the latter study showed that durvalumab has activity against pancreatic cancer, the discouraging response rates of immune checkpoint inhibitors in the treatment of pancreatic cancer from multiple studies warrant further preclinical and clinical research. Designing an appropriate combination treatment regimen that can overcome the immunosuppressive tumor microenvironment of pancreatic cancer can be one of the keys to improving the efficacy of immunotherapy. For example, given its immune modulatory effects, acalabrutinib, a tyrosine kinase inhibitor, has recently been tested in pancreatic cancer in combination with pembrolizumab (NCT02362048) (Overman et al. 2016).

Colorectal Cancer

Metastatic colorectal cancer (mCRC) is a significant cause of mortality and morbidity in the USA. Approximately 25–30% of patients with newly diagnosed CRC have evidence of metastases upon diagnosis (Cancer.org). Its treatment outcome has been significantly improved over the last decade with the incorporation of biological targeted therapies to systemic chemotherapies. However, therapy resistance remains a clinical challenge. Immunotherapy approaches have recently been explored in the treatment of mCRC in order to further improve the outcomes.

Deficient DNA mismatch repair (dMMR) has been identified in approximately 15–20% of sporadic CRC and in patients with Lynch syndrome, resulting in high levels of DNA replication errors and DNA microsatellite instability (MSI) than those of proficient MMR (pMMR). These tumors harbor greater mutational burdens, therefore more neoantigens are presented to tumor-specific T cells that can target tumor cells for killing. Immune checkpoint inhibitors can unleash the functions of these T cells and potentially improve the anti-tumor activities. Multiple clinical trials have demonstrated clear efficacy of PD-1 inhibitors in a subset of mCRC patients.

Pembrolizumab, an anti-PD-1 antibody, was evaluated in a phase 2 study enrolling 28 patients with dMMR CRCs and 25 patients with pMMR CRCs (Le et al. 2016). The ORR was 50% in the dMMR group versus 0% in the pMMR group, and the DCR was 89% and 16% in the dMMR and pMMR groups, respectively. For patients with dMMR disease, the 24-month OS was 66% and the 24-month PFS was 61%. The toxicity profile was comparable to other reported trials with pembrolizumab monotherapy. These data led to the FDA granting accelerated approval of pembrolizumab for patients with advanced MSI-High (MSI-H) or dMMR mCRC who have progressed after conventional chemotherapy.

Nivolumab was also tested in patients with dMMR mCRC in a phase 2 trial (Overman et al. 2017). Among 74 patients who received nivolumab monotherapy at 3 mg/kg every 2 weeks, 31% had an objective response, and the median duration of response was not reached with a median follow-up of 12 months. In addition, the responses were observed regardless of BRAF or KRAS mutation status.

Despite these encouraging results, anti-PD-1 antibodies provide low response rates in mCRC patients with proficient MMR and microsatellite stable (MSS) tumors, which represent the vast majority of patients. Further clinical trials have been designed to examine the combination therapy strategies for pMMR and MSS mCRCs. Atezolizumab, a PD-L1 inhibitor, in combination with cobimetinib, a MEK kinase inhibitor, was investigated in a recent phase 1 trial (Bendell et al. 2016). A total of 23 patients were enrolled, of which 22 were KRAS mutant. The preliminary results showed an ORR of 17% (four out of 23 patients), and three out of the four responders have pMMR tumors. This study provides evidence supporting further investigations of alternative immunotherapy strategies for MSS mCRCs.

Anal squamous cell carcinoma (SCC) is commonly associated with infection by the human papillomavirus (HPV). Other conditions, such as immune inhibition, are also known risk factors (Palefsky et al. 2011). The potential role of PD-1 blockade in the treatment of anal SCC was examined in recent trials. In a phase 2 clinical study (NCT02314169) (Morris et al. 2017), nivolumab was given to a total of 37 HPV+ patients, and 24% had a response. The median OS and PFS were 11.5 months and 4.1 months, respectively.

Head and Neck Cancer

Head and neck squamous cell carcinoma (HNSCC) is the sixth most common malignancy in the world. In addition to tobacco and alcohol use as known risk factors, human HPVs are associated with a subset of HNSCCs with distinct clinical features, including a better treatment response and prognosis. Although multimodality treatment strategies have advanced over the past decade, the prognosis and survival for patients with recurrent or metastatic HNSCC remain poor, underscoring the necessity of developing novel therapeutic strategies, including immunotherapy.

The efficacy of pembrolizumab in HNSCC has been established in multiple clinical trials, which led to the FDA approval for platinum-refractory metastatic or recurrent HNSCC. In the KEYNOTE-012 expansion cohort, 132 patients irrespective of PD-L1 or HPV status were enrolled and received pembrolizumab once every 3 weeks. ORR was 18% with a median duration of response that was not reached. Six-month PFS was 23% and 6-month OS was 59%. In the KEYNOTE-055 study, 171 platinum- and cetuximab-refractory HNSCC patients received pembrolizumab. The ORR was 16% in this study with a median duration of response of 8 months. The median PFS was 2.1 months and median OS was 8 months. Eighty-two percent of patients had PD-L1 positive tumors while 22% were HPV positive. Interestingly, the response rate was similar in all HPV and PD-L1 subgroups. Phase 3 trials with pembrolizumab are currently underway (NCT02252042).

The CheckMate 141 phase 3 trial randomized patients to either nivolumab or a single-agent therapy of the investigator's choice (Ferris et al. 2016). A total of 361 platinum-refractory recurrent or metastatic HNSCC patients were enrolled, and median follow-up was 5.1 months. For the entire study population, OS was significantly longer in the nivolumab group (median 7.5 vs. 5.1 months), and the ORR was also increased in the nivolumab group (13.3% vs. 5.8%). In patients with PD-L1+ tumors ($\geq 1\%$), OS was significantly improved with nivolumab (8.7 vs. 4.6 months), but was not increased in patients with less than 1% PD-L1 expression tumors. In addition, OS was also significantly improved with nivolumab in HPV-positive tumors but not in HPV-negative tumors. Nivolumab was granted approval by the FDA based on these results.

Despite the promising results from the abovementioned trials, the majority of patients do not benefit from anti-PD1 monotherapy, highlighting the need to develop alternative immunotherapy strategies to improve the overall outcomes. Multiple clinical trials are designed and currently ongoing to evaluate the combination approaches. For example, the efficacy of durvalumab, a PD-L1 inhibitor, alone or in combination with tremelimumab, a CTLA-4 inhibitor, versus chemotherapy is currently being assessed in a phase 3 trial (NCT02369874) in patients with previously treated recurrent and metastatic HNSCC. Durvalumab alone or in combination with tremlimumab is also being investigated for first-line treatment in recurrent or metastatic HNSCC in the phase 3 KESTREL study (NCT02551159). The anti-tumor activity of durvalumab monotherapy in PD-L1-positive HNSCC was previously demonstrated in early studies (Fury et al. 2014; Segal et al. 2016).

Other Solid Tumors

Given the rapid advances in tumor immunotherapy and promising results from clinical studies that led to the FDA approval of immune checkpoint inhibitors, such treatment strategies have been actively investigated in and expanded to multiple other types of malignancies. Although most of these results have yet to be confirmed in further clinical trials, these novel agents are rapidly changing the landscape of cancer therapy. Most of the FDA-approved indications of immune checkpoint inhibitors have already been discussed in detail in other chapters in this book. In this section, we briefly review their roles in gynecologic malignancies and Merkel cell carcinoma, which have been recently investigated in clinical trials. The utilization of immune checkpoint inhibitors in many solid tumors is still being clinically investigated and is only available through clinical trials. Since the field of immunotherapy is rapidly evolving and results of clinical trials are constantly being reported, we are not able to review all of the trials in all of the tumor types and their corresponding results here. For the most updated list, we would like to refer readers to https://clinicaltrials.gov for further information. We strongly recommend open discussions between patients and oncologists to explore the most updated results from clinical research and ongoing clinical trial options before formulating personalized treatment strategies.

Recurrent or metastatic gynecologic malignancies are associated with great morbidity and mortality in females. Immune checkpoint inhibitors have been recently adapted for the management of cervical, ovarian, and endometrial cancers; however, none of them have yet gained approval from the FDA.

Although HPV vaccination can provide protection against cervical cancer, the available treatment options for recurrent or advanced disease are very limited. In the KEYNOTE-028 study, advanced cervical cancer patients with PD-L1 positive tumors were treated with pembrolizumab (anti-PD-1 antibody). In 24 treated patients, an ORR of 12.5% was observed (Frenel et al. 2016). The preliminary results from the phase 2 KEYNOTE-158 study later reported an ORR of 17% in patients with previously treated cervical cancer unselective for PD-L1 expression status (Schellens et al. 2017).

Advanced endometrial cancer carries a poor prognosis, and is traditionally treated with chemotherapy. Defects in DNA mismatch repair machinery (dMMR) and resultant microsatellite instability (MSI) status (as previously discussed in the metastatic colon cancer section) are found in approximately 20% of tumors from endometrial cancer patients, which suggests a potential role of immunotherapy in this tumor type. In a recently reported phase 2 trial, pembrolizumab demonstrated an ORR of 71% in MSI-high non-colorectal malignancies, including two patients with endometrial cancer (one with partial response, and one with complete response) (Le et al. 2015). The safety and anti-tumor activity of pembrolizumab in advanced endometrial cancer patients who have positive PD-L1 expression were also tested in the KEYNOTE-028 study (Ott et al. 2017). Three out of the 24 treated patients experienced a partial response and three patients had stable diseases. Multiple ongoing studies are underway to explore the roles of combination therapies, including with chemotherapy (e.g., NCT02549209 and NCT02331251 for pembrolizumab with chemotherapy) and immunotherapy (NCT02982486 for nivolumab with immunotherapy).

In patients with platinum-resistant advanced ovarian cancer, antibodies against PD-L1 (avelumab) and PD-1 (nivolumab and pembrolizumab) have been tested in early-phase clinical studies (Disis et al. 2016). In NCT01772004, avelumab was reported to have an ORR of 9.7%. In a study using pembrolizumab (NCT02054806) (Varga et al. 2015), patients with positive PD-L1 status showed an ORR of 11.5%. Nivolumab was also reported to have an ORR of 15% in a study with 20 patients (Hamanishi et al. 2015). In the light of the low response rates of single PD-1/PD-L1 blockade, currently ongoing clinical trials are focused on investigating the safety and efficacy of immunotherapy combined with molecular-targeted therapy, chemotherapy, or immunotherapy. For example, olaparib, a polyadenosine diphosphate-ribose polymerase (PARP) inhibitor that was approved for the treatment of recurrent/metastatic ovarian cancer, has been combined with durvalumab (PD-L1 antibody) in patients with BRCA mutations. Preliminary results from this trial demonstrated an ORR of 17% with a high disease control rate (83%) (Lee et al. 2017). Pembrolizumab is being investigated in combination with chemotherapies (e.g., paclitaxel, gemcitabine, and cisplatin) in clinical trials (NCT02440425, NCT02608684). Avelumab combined with doxil is being tested in NCT02580058. The combination of nivolumab with ipilimumab is being examined in the CheckMate 032 study (NCT01928394).

Merkel cell carcinoma is (MCC) an aggressive cutaneous malignancy with a tendency to recurrence and metastases. Given the rarity of this disease, few randomized clinical trials have been reported to establish the effective treatment regimens for metastatic disease, although cytotoxic chemotherapy approaches have been the standard-of-care for years. Recently, immune checkpoint inhibitors have been shown to be a potential alternative. Avelumab was recently approved by the FDA for the treatment of previously treated metastatic MCC based on the phase 2 JAVELIN Merkel 200 trial. A total of 88 patients were enrolled in this study, and 28 had objective responses, including eight complete responses. The 6-month PFS and OS were 40% and 69%, respectively, suggesting a durable response. Infusion-related reactions were observed in 17% of the patients; fortunately, they are all low-grade and easily managed with supportive measures (Kaufman et al. 2016). It is otherwise well tolerated. Pembrolizumab was also reported to be effective in the treatment of advanced MCC in a phase 2 study (Nghiem et al. 2016). A total of 26 patients who had not received previous systemic therapy were enrolled, and an ORR of 56% was reported with a 6-month PFS of 67%, indicating its potential role in front-line settings.

Biomarker Considerations

One of the main challenges in the field of cancer immunotherapy is the development of reliable predictive and prognostic biomarkers, which can guide the best selection of patients who will benefit from such a treatment modality and provide early prediction of disease response while on therapy. Several candidate biomarkers have been investigated, including PD-L1 expression level and MMR/MSI status.

The utilization and limitation of PD-L expression levels as a potential biomarker has been discussed in Chapter 4, "Significance of Immune Checkpoints in Lung Cancer." Its level has been associated with a better clinical response with antibodies targeting the PD-1/PD-L1 pathway in some of the studies. For example, in a study reported in 2012, nivolumab was studied in patients with advanced solid tumors, including melanoma, lung cancer, and colorectal cancer. In that study, nine out of 25 patients with PD-L1 expression responded to the therapy, while none (0/17) of the patients with PD-L1-negative tumors responded to the treatment (Topalian et al. 2012). However, in other studies, patients with PD-L1-negative tumors also demonstrated responses towards anti-PD-1 therapy (Weber et al. 2015; Brahmer et al. 2015). These inconsistent results indicate that PD-L1 expression is an imperfect surrogate and predictor for immunological and therapeutic response, and its role in clinical practice is still investigational and under debate. The levels of PD-L1 expression from tumor biopsies under-represent the complex, dynamic, and heterogeneous tumor microenvironment. In addition, the test methodology, the platform used in clinical practice, and the agreement between different tests need further validations across various tumor types. Tumor PD-L1 expression should not be simply used to exclude patients with advanced cancer from being considered to receive immunotherapy.

As we previously discussed in Section 2.5 (Colorectal Cancer), preclinical research has demonstrated that tumors that are defective in DNA mismatch repair genes (dMMR) have higher levels of microsatellite instability, and therefore carry a higher mutational burden, which results in a greater level of neo-antigens that can be recognized by tumor-specific T cells exerting the anti-tumor activities. The frequency of dMMR or MSI-H tumors are reported to be around 15–20% in sporadic CRC, 8–16% in gastric cancer, and 25% in endometrial cancerf (An et al. 2012; Howitt et al. 2015). The role of dMMR/MSI-H as a biomarker for clinical response to PD-1 blockade has been recently established in a clinical trial that included patients with 12 different types of solid tumors that are dMMR. Among 86 patients who received pembrolizumab, 53% achieved an objective response with 21% achieving a complete response (Lee et al. 2017). Clinical data from 149 patients with dMMR or MSI-H cancers enrolled across five single-arm KEYNOTE trials (KEYNOTE-016, −164, −012, −028, and −158) have led to the recently accelerated FDA approval of pembrolizumab for adult and pediatric patients with unresected or metastatic dMMR or MSI-H solid tumors that have progressed following previous treatment with no satisfactory alternative treatment options. The reported ORR was 39.6%, with 7.4% having a complete response and 78% of the responders had responses that lasted for more than 6 months. This is the first FDA approval of cancer therapy based on biomarkers regardless of tumor type.

Conclusion

Immune checkpoint inhibitors are rapidly changing the paradigm of cancer treatments. Continued research efforts are needed to design more effective and individualized treatment regimens for various types of malignancies. In addition, identification of patients who will benefit from treatment, development of reliable biomarkers, and minimizing the treatment toxicities will remain an active focus of research.

References

Ali, H. R., Provenzano, E., Dawson, S. J., Blows, F. M., Liu, B., Shah, M., Earl, H. M., Poole, C. J., Hiller, L., Dunn, J. A., Bowden, S. J., Twelves, C., Bartlett, J. M., Mahmoud, S. M., Rakha, E., Ellis, I. O., Liu, S., Gao, D., Nielsen, T. O., Pharoah, P. D., & Caldas, C. (2014). Association between CD8+ T-cell infiltration and breast cancer survival in 12,439 patients. *Annals of Oncology, 25,* 1536–1543.

Ali, H. R., Glont, S. E., Blows, F. M., Provenzano, E., Dawson, S. J., Liu, B., Hiller, L., Dunn, J., Poole, C. J., Bowden, S., Earl, H. M., Pharoah, P. D., & Caldas, C. (2015). PD-L1 protein expression in breast cancer is rare, enriched in basal-like tumours and associated with infiltrating lymphocytes. *Annals of Oncology, 26,* 1488–1493.

An, J. Y., Kim, H., Cheong, J. H., Hyung, W. J., Kim, H., & Noh, S. H. (2012). Microsatellite instability in sporadic gastric cancer: Its prognostic role and guidance for 5-FU based chemotherapy after R0 resection. *International Journal of Cancer, 131,* 505–511.

Bang, Y. J., Doi, T., De Braud, F., Piha-Paul, S., Hollebecque, A., Razak, A. R. A., Lin, C. C., Ott, P. A., He, A. R., Yuan, S. S., Koshiji, M., Lam, B., & Aggarwal, R. (2015). Safety and efficacy of pembrolizumab (MK-3475) in patients (pts) with advanced biliary tract cancer: Interim results of KEYNOTE-028. *European Journal of Cancer, 51,* S112–S112.

Bendell, J. C., Kim, T. W., Goh, B. C., Wallin, J., Oh, D. Y., Han, S. W., Lee, C. B., Hellmann, M. D., Desai, J., Lewin, J. H., Solomon, B. J., Chow, L. Q. M., Miller, W. H., Gainor, J. F., Flaherty, K., Infante, J. R., Das-Thakur, M., Foster, P., Cha, E., & Bang, Y. J. (2016). Clinical activity and safety of cobimetinib (cobi) and atezolizumab in colorectal cancer (CRC). *Journal of Clinical Oncology, 34*(36), 4307–4453.

Brahmer, J. R., Tykodi, S. S., Chow, L. Q., Hwu, W. J., Topalian, S. L., Hwu, P., Drake, C. G., Camacho, L. H., Kauh, J., Odunsi, K., Pitot, H. C., Hamid, O., Bhatia, S., Martins, R., Eaton, K., Chen, S., Salay, T. M., Alaparthy, S., Grosso, J. F., Korman, A. J., Parker, S. M., Agrawal, S., Goldberg, S. M., Pardoll, D. M., Gupta, A., & Wigginton, J. M. (2012). Safety and activity of anti-PD-L1 antibody in patients with advanced cancer. *The New England Journal of Medicine, 366,* 2455–2465.

Brahmer, J., Reckamp, K. L., Baas, P., Crino, L., Eberhardt, W. E., Poddubskaya, E., Antonia, S., Pluzanski, A., Vokes, E. E., Holgado, E., Waterhouse, D., Ready, N., Gainor, J., Aren Frontera, O., Havel, L., Steins, M., Garassino, M. C., Aerts, J. G., Domine, M., PAZ-ARES, L., RECK, M., Baudelet, C., Harbison, C. T., Lestini, B., & Spigel, D. R. (2015). Nivolumab versus docetaxel in advanced squamous-cell non-small-cell lung cancer. *The New England Journal of Medicine, 373,* 123–135.

Cancer.Org. (2017). Cancer estimates.

Cancer.Org. *American Cancer Society.*

Crocenzi, T. S., El-Khoueiry, A. B., & Cheung, T. (2017). Nivolumab (nivo) in sorafenib (sor)-naive and -experienced pts with advanced hepatocellular carcinoma (HCC): CheckMate 040 study. *Journal of Clinical Oncology, 35,* 3541–3543.

Denkert, C., Loibl, S., Noske, A., Roller, M., Muller, B. M., Komor, M., Budczies, J., Darb-Esfahani, S., Kronenwett, R., Hanusch, C., Von Torne, C., Weichert, W., Engels, K., Solbach, C., Schrader, I., Dietel, M., & Von Minckwitz, G. (2010). Tumor-associated lymphocytes as an independent predictor of response to neoadjuvant chemotherapy in breast cancer. *Journal of Clinical Oncology, 28*, 105–113.

Derks, S., Liao, X., Chiaravalli, A. M., Xu, X., Camargo, M. C., Solcia, E., Sessa, F., Fleitas, T., Freeman, G. J., Rodig, S. J., Rabkin, C. S., & Bass, A. J. (2016). Abundant PD-L1 expression in epstein-barr virus-infected gastric cancers. *Oncotarget, 7*, 32925–32932.

Dirix, L. Y., Takacs, I., Nikolinakos, P., Jerusalem, G., Arkenau, H. T., Hamilton, E. P., Von Heydebreck, A., Grote, H. J., Chin, K., & Lippman, M. E. (2016). Avelumab (MSB0010718C), an anti-PD-L1 antibody, in patients with locally advanced or metastatic breast cancer: A phase 1b JAVELIN solid tumor trial. *Cancer Research, 76*(4 Supplement), Abstract S1–04.

Disis, M. L., Patel, M. R., Pant, S., Hamilton, E. P., Lockhart, A. C., Kelly, K., Beck, J. T., Gordon, M. S., Weiss, G. J., Taylor, M. H., Chaves, J., Mita, A. C., Chin, K. M., Von Heydebreck, A., Cuillerot, J. M., & Gulley, J. L. (2016). Avelumab (MSB0010718C; anti-PD-L1) in patients with recurrent/refractory ovarian cancer from the JAVELIN Solid Tumor phase Ib trial: Safety and clinical activity. *Journal of Clinical Oncology, 34*(15_suppl), 5533.

Doi, T., Piha-Paul, S. A., Jalal, S. I., Mai-Dang, H., Yuan, S., Koshiji, M., Csiki, I., & Bennouna, J. (2015). Pembrolizumab (MK-3475) for patients (pts) with advanced esophageal carcinoma: Preliminary results from KEYNOTE-028. *Journal of Clinical Oncology, 33*(15_suppl), 4010.

El-Khoueiry, A. B., Sangro, B., Yau, T., Crocenzi, T. S., Kudo, M., Hsu, C., Kim, T. Y., Choo, S. P., Trojan, J., Welling, T. H. R., Meyer, T., Kang, Y. K., Yeo, W., Chopra, A., Anderson, J., Dela Cruz, C., Lang, L., Neely, J., Tang, H., Dastani, H. B., & Melero, I. (2017). Nivolumab in patients with advanced hepatocellular carcinoma (CheckMate 040): An open-label, non-comparative, phase 1/2 dose escalation and expansion trial. *Lancet, 389*, 2492–2502.

Emens, L. A., Braiteh, F., Cassier, P. A., Delord, J. P., Eder, J. P., & Fasso, M. (2015). Inhibition of PD-L1 by MPDL3280A leads to clinical activity in patients with metastatic triple-negative breast cancer (TNBC). *Cancer Research, 75*(15 Supplement), abstract 2859.

Ferlay, J., Soerjomataram, I., Dikshit, R., Eser, S., Mathers, C., Rebelo, M., Parkin, D. M., Forman, D., & Bray, F. (2015). Cancer incidence and mortality worldwide: Sources, methods and major patterns in GLOBOCAN 2012. *International Journal of Cancer, 136*, E359–E386.

Ferris, R. L., Blumenschein, G., Jr., Fayette, J., Guigay, J., Colevas, A. D., Licitra, L., Harrington, K., Kasper, S., Vokes, E. E., Even, C., Worden, F., Saba, N. F., Iglesias Docampo, L. C., Haddad, R., Rordorf, T., Kiyota, N., Tahara, M., Monga, M., Lynch, M., Geese, W. J., Kopit, J., Shaw, J. W., & Gillison, M. L. (2016). Nivolumab for recurrent squamous-cell carcinoma of the head and neck. *The New England Journal of Medicine, 375*, 1856–1867.

Frenel, J. S., Le Tourneau, C., O'neil, B. H., Ott, P. A., Piha-Paul, S. A., Gomez-Roca, C. A., Van Brummelen, E., Rugo, H. S., Thomas, S., Saraf, S., Chen, M., & Varga, A. (2016). Pembrolizumab in patients with advanced cervical squamous cell cancer: Preliminary results from the phase Ib KEYNOTE-028 study. *Journal of Clinical Oncology, 34*(15_suppl), 5515.

Fuchs, C. S., Doi, T., Jang, R. W.-J., Muro, K., Satoh, T., Machado, M., Sun, W., Jalal, S. I., Shah, M. A., Metges, J.-P., Garrido, M., Golan, T., mandala, m., Wainberg, Z. A., Catenacci, D. V. T., Bang, Y.-J., Wang, J., Koshiji, M., Dalal, R. P., & Yoon, H. H. (2017). KEYNOTE-059 cohort 1: Efficacy and safety of pembrolizumab (pembro) monotherapy in patients with previously treated advanced gastric cancer. *ASCO, 35*(31), 3519–3634.

Fury, M.,Butler, M., Ou, S., Balmanoukian, A., et al. (2014). Clinical activity and safety of MEDI4736, an anti-PD-L1 antibody, in head and neck cancer. *ESMO Meeting 2014,* Poster No 988PD.

Gani, F., Nagarajan, N., Kim, Y., Zhu, Q., Luan, L., Bhaijjee, F., Anders, R. A., & Pawlik, T. M. (2016). Program death 1 immune checkpoint and tumor microenvironment: Implications for patients with intrahepatic cholangiocarcinoma. *Annals of Surgical Oncology, 23*, 2610–2617.

Gao, Q., Wang, X. Y., Qiu, S. J., Yamato, I., Sho, M., Nakajima, Y., Zhou, J., Li, B. Z., Shi, Y. H., Xiao, Y. S., Xu, Y., & Fan, J. (2009). Overexpression of PD-L1 significantly associates with tumor aggressiveness and postoperative recurrence in human hepatocellular carcinoma. *Clinical Cancer Research, 15*, 971–979.

Hamanishi, J., Mandai, M., Ikeda, T., Minami, M., Kawaguchi, A., Murayama, T., Kanai, M., Mori, Y., Matsumoto, S., Chikuma, S., Matsumura, N., Abiko, K., Baba, T., Yamaguchi, K., Ueda, A., Hosoe, Y., Morita, S., Yokode, M., Shimizu, A., Honjo, T., & Konishi, I. (2015). Safety and antitumor activity of anti-PD-1 antibody, nivolumab, in patients with platinum-resistant ovarian cancer. *Journal of Clinical Oncology, 33*, 4015–4022.

Howitt, B. E., Shukla, S. A., Sholl, L. M., Ritterhouse, L. L., Watkins, J. C., Rodig, S., Stover, E., Strickland, K. C., D'andrea, A. D., Wu, C. J., Matulonis, U. A., & Konstantinopoulos, P. A. (2015). Association of Polymerase e-Mutated and Microsatellite-Instable Endometrial Cancers with Neoantigen Load, Number of Tumor-Infiltrating Lymphocytes, and Expression of PD-1 and PD-L1. *JAMA Oncology, 1*, 1319–1323.

Kang, Y.-K., Satoh, T., Ryu, M.-H., Chao, Y., Kato, K., Chung, H. C., Chen, J.-S., Muro, K., Kang, W. K., & Yoshikawa, T. (2017). Nivolumab (ONO-4538/BMS-936558) as salvage treatment after second or later-line chemotherapy for advanced gastric or gastro-esophageal junction cancer (AGC): A double-blinded, randomized,phase III trial. *Journal of Clinical Oncology, 35*, 2–2.

Kaufman, H. L., Russell, J., Hamid, O., Bhatia, S., Terheyden, P., D'angelo, S. P., Shih, K. C., Lebbe, C., Linette, G. P., Milella, M., Brownell, I., Lewis, K. D., Lorch, J. H., Chin, K., Mahnke, L., Von Heydebreck, A., Cuillerot, J. M., & Nghiem, P. (2016). Avelumab in patients with chemotherapy-refractory metastatic Merkel cell carcinoma: A multicentre, single-group, open-label, phase 2 trial. *The Lancet Oncology, 17*, 1374–1385.

Kudo, T., Hamamoto, Y., Kato, K., Ura, T., Kojima, T., Tsushima, T., Hironaka, S., Hara, H., Satoh, T., Iwasa, S., Muro, K., Yasui, H., Minashi, K., Yamaguchi, K., Ohtsu, A., Doki, Y., & Kitagawa, Y. (2017). Nivolumab treatment for oesophageal squamous-cell carcinoma: An open-label, multicentre, phase 2 trial. *The Lancet Oncology, 18*, 631–639.

Lawrence, M. S., Stojanov, P., Polak, P., Kryukov, G. V., Cibulskis, K., Sivachenko, A., Carter, S. L., Stewart, C., Mermel, C. H., Roberts, S. A., Kiezun, A., Hammerman, P. S., Mckenna, A., Drier, Y., Zou, L., Ramos, A. H., Pugh, T. J., Stransky, N., Helman, E., Kim, J., Sougnez, C., Ambrogio, L., Nickerson, E., Shefler, E., Cortes, M. L., Auclair, D., Saksena, G., Voet, D., Noble, M., Dicara, D., Lin, P., Lichtenstein, L., Heiman, D. I., Fennell, T., Imielinski, M., Hernandez, B., Hodis, E., Baca, S., Dulak, A. M., Lohr, J., Landau, D. A., Wu, C. J., Melendez-Zajgla, J., Hidalgo-Miranda, A., Koren, A., Mccarroll, S. A., Mora, J., Crompton, B., Onofrio, R., Parkin, M., Winckler, W., Ardlie, K., Gabriel, S. B., Roberts, C. W. M., Biegel, J. A., Stegmaier, K., Bass, A. J., Garraway, L. A., Meyerson, M., Golub, T. R., Gordenin, D. A., Sunyaev, S., Lander, E. S., & Getz, G. (2013). Mutational heterogeneity in cancer and the search for new cancer-associated genes. *Nature, 499*, 214–218.

Le, D. T., Uram, J. N., Wang, H., Bartlett, B. R., Kemberling, H., Eyring, A. D., Skora, A. D., Luber, B. S., Azad, N. S., Laheru, D., Biedrzycki, B., Donehower, R. C., Zaheer, A., Fisher, G. A., Crocenzi, T. S., Lee, J. J., Duffy, S. M., Goldberg, R. M., De La Chapelle, A., Koshiji, M., Bhaijee, F., Huebner, T., Hruban, R. H., Wood, L. D., Cuka, N., Pardoll, D. M., Papadopoulos, N., Kinzler, K. W., Zhou, S., Cornish, T. C., Taube, J. M., Anders, R. A., Eshleman, J. R., Vogelstein, B., & Diaz, L. A., Jr. (2015). PD-1 blockade in tumors with mismatch-repair deficiency. *The New England Journal of Medicine, 372*, 2509–2520.

Le, D. T., Uram, J. N., Wang, H., Bartlett, B., Kemberling, H., Eyring, A., Azad, N. S., Laheru, D., Donehower, R. C., Crocenzi, T. S., Goldberg, R. M., Fisher, G. A., Lee, J. J., Greten, T. F., Koshiji, M., Kang, S. P., Anders, R. A., Eshleman, J. R., Vogelstein, B., & Diaz, L. A. (2016). Programmed death-1 blockade in mismatch repair deficient colorectal cancer. *Journal of Clinical Oncology, 34*(15_suppl), 103.

Le, D. T., Durham, J. N., Smith, K. N., Wang, H., Bartlett, B. R., Aulakh, L. K., Lu, S., Kemberling, H., Wilt, C., Luber, B. S., Wong, F., Azad, N. S., Rucki, A. A., Laheru, D., Donehower, R., Zaheer, A., Fisher, G. A., Crocenzi, T. S., Lee, J. J., Greten, T. F., Duffy, A. G., Ciombor, K. K., Eyring, A. D., Lam, B. H., Joe, A., Kang, S. P., Holdhoff, M., Danilova, L., Cope, L., Meyer, C., Zhou, S., Goldberg, R. M., Armstrong, D. K., Bever, K. M., Fader, A. N., Taube, J., Housseau, F., Spetzler, D., Xiao, N., Pardoll, D. M., Papadopoulos, N., Kinzler, K. W., Eshleman, J. R., Vogelstein, B., Anders, R. A., & Diaz, L. A., Jr. (2017). Mismatch repair deficiency predicts response of solid tumors to PD-1 blockade. *Science, 357*, 409–413.

Lee, J. M., Cimino-Mathews, A., Peer, C. J., Zimmer, A., Lipkowitz, S., Annunziata, C. M., CAO, L., Harrell, M. I., Swisher, E., Houston, N., Botesteanu, D. A., Taube, J. M., Thompson, E., Ogurtsova, A., Xu, H. Y., Nguyen, J., Ho, T. W., Figg, W. D., & Kohn, E. C. (2017). Safety and clinical activity of the programmed death-ligand 1 inhibitor durvalumab in combination with poly (ADP-Ribose) polymerase inhibitor olaparib or vascular endothelial growth factor receptor 1-3 inhibitor cediranib in women's cancers: A dose-escalation, phase I study. *Journal of Clinical Oncology, 35,* 2193.

Liu, Y. X., Wang, X. S., Wang, Y. F., Hu, X. C., Yan, J. Q., Zhang, Y. L., Wang, W., Yang, R. J., Feng, Y. Y., GAO, S. G., & FENG, X. S. (2016). Prognostic significance of PD-L1 expression in patients with gastric cancer in East Asia: A meta-analysis. *Oncotargets and Therapy, 9,* 2649–2654.

Morris, V. K., Salem, M. E., Nimeiri, H., Iqbal, S., Singh, P., Ciombor, K., Polite, B., Deming, D., Chan, E., Wade, J. L., Xiao, L. C., Bekaii-Saab, T., Vence, L., Blando, J., Mahvash, A., Foo, W. C., Ohaji, C., Pasia, M., Bland, G., Ohinata, A., Rogers, J., Mehdizadeh, A., Banks, K., Lanman, R., Wolff, R. A., Streicher, H., Allison, J., Sharma, P., & Eng, C. (2017). Nivolumab for previously treated unresectable metastatic anal cancer (NCI9673): A multicentre, single-arm, phase 2 study. *The Lancet Oncology, 18,* 446–453.

Muro, K., Chung, H. C., Shankaran, V., Geva, R., Catenacci, D., Gupta, S., Eder, J. P., Golan, T., Le, D. T., Burtness, B., Mcree, A. J., Lin, C. C., Pathiraja, K., Lunceford, J., Emancipator, K., Juco, J., Koshiji, M., & Bang, Y. J. (2016). Pembrolizumab for patients with PD-L1-positive advanced gastric cancer (KEYNOTE-012): A multicentre, open-label, phase 1b trial. *The Lancet Oncology, 17,* 717–726.

Nanda, R., Chow, L. Q., Dees, E. C., Berger, R., Gupta, S., Geva, R., Pusztai, L., Pathiraja, K., Aktan, G., Cheng, J. D., Karantza, V., & Buisseret, L. (2016). Pembrolizumab in patients with advanced triple-negative breast cancer: Phase Ib KEYNOTE-012 study. *Journal of Clinical Oncology, 34,* 2460–2467.

Nghiem, P. T., Bhatia, S., Lipson, E. J., Kudchadkar, R. R., Miller, N. J., Annamalai, L., Berry, S., Chartash, E. K., Daud, A., Fling, S. P., Friedlander, P. A., Kluger, H. M., Kohrt, H. E., Lundgren, L., MARGOLIN, K., MITCHELL, A., Olencki, T., Pardoll, D. M., Reddy, S. A., Shantha, E. M., Sharfman, W. H., Sharon, E., Shemanski, L. R., Shinohara, M. M., Sunshine, J. C., Taube, J. M., Thompson, J. A., Townson, S. M., Yearley, J. H., Topalian, S. L., & Cheever, M. A. (2016). PD-1 blockade with pembrolizumab in advanced merkel-cell carcinoma. *The New England Journal of Medicine, 374,* 2542–2552.

Ohigashi, Y., Sho, M., Yamada, Y., Tsurui, Y., Hamada, K., Ikeda, N., Mizuno, T., Yoriki, R., Kashizuka, H., Yane, K., Tsushima, F., Otsuki, N., Yagita, H., Azuma, M., & Nakajima, Y. (2005). Clinical significance of programmed death-1 ligand-1 and programmed death-1 ligand-2 expression in human esophageal cancer. *Clinical Cancer Research, 11,* 2947–2953.

Ott, P. A., Bang, Y. J., Berton-Rigaud, D., Elez, E., Pishvaian, M. J., Rugo, H. S., Puzanov, I., Mehnert, J. M., Aung, K. L., Lopez, J., Carrigan, M., Saraf, S., Chen, M., & Soria, J. C. (2017). Safety and antitumor activity of pembrolizumab in advanced programmed death ligand 1-positive endometrial cancer: Results from the KEYNOTE-028 study. *Journal of Clinical Oncology, 35,* 2535–2541.

Overman, M. J., Lopez, C. D., Benson, A., Neelapu, S. S., Mettu, N. B., Ko, A. H., Chung, V. M., Nemunaitis, J. J., Reeves, J. A., Bendell, J. C., Philip, P. A., Dalal, R., Fardis, M., Greer, J., Wang, X. L., Inamdar, S., Lannutti, B. J., Rothbaum, W., Izumi, R., & Javle, M. M. (2016). A randomized phase 2 study of the Bruton tyrosine kinase (Btk) inhibitor acalabrutinib alone or with pembrolizumab for metastatic pancreatic cancer (mPC). *Journal of Clinical Oncology, 34*(15_suppl), 4130.

Overman, M. J., Mcdermott, R., Leach, J. L., Lonardi, S., Lenz, H. J., Morse, M. A., Desai, J., Hill, A., Axelson, M., Moss, R. A., Goldberg, M. V., Cao, Z. A., Ledeine, J. M., Maglinte, G. A., Kopetz, S., & Andre, T. (2017). Nivolumab in patients with metastatic DNA mismatch repair-deficient or microsatellite instability-high colorectal cancer (CheckMate 142): An open-label, multicentre, phase 2 study. *The Lancet Oncology, 18,* 1182–1191.

Palefsky, J. M., Giuliano, A. R., Goldstone, S., Moreira, E. D., Aranda, C., Jessen, H., Hillman, R., Ferris, D., Coutlee, F., Stoler, M. H., Marshall, J. B., Radley, D., Vuocolo, S., Haupt, R. M., Guris, D., & Garner, E. I. O. (2011). HPV Vaccine against anal HPV infection and anal intraepithelial neoplasia. *The New England Journal of Medicine, 365*, 1576–1585.

Rizvi, N. A., Hellmann, M. D., Snyder, A., Kvistborg, P., Makarov, V., Havel, J. J., Lee, W., Yuan, J., Wong, P., Ho, T. S., Miller, M. L., Rekhtman, N., Moreira, A. L., Ibrahim, F., Bruggeman, C., Gasmi, B., Zappasodi, R., Maeda, Y., Sander, C., Garon, E. B., Merghoub, T., Wolchok, J. D., Schumacher, T. N., & Chan, T. A. (2015). Cancer immunology. Mutational landscape determines sensitivity to PD-1 blockade in non-small cell lung cancer. *Science, 348*, 124–128.

Royal, R. E., Levy, C., Turner, K., Mathur, A., Hughes, M., Kammula, U. S., Sherry, R. M., Topalian, S. L., Yang, J. C., Lowy, I., & Rosenberg, S. A. (2010). Phase 2 trial of single agent Ipilimumab (anti-CTLA-4) for locally advanced or metastatic pancreatic adenocarcinoma. *Journal of Immunotherapy, 33*, 828–833.

Sabatier, R., Finetti, P., Mamessier, E., Adelaide, J., Chaffanet, M., Ali, H. R., Viens, P., Caldas, C., Birnbaum, D., & Bertucci, F. (2015). Prognostic and predictive value of PDL1 expression in breast cancer. *Oncotarget, 6*, 5449–5464.

Salgado, R., Denkert, C., Demaria, S., Sirtaine, N., Klauschen, F., Pruneri, G., Wienert, S., Van Den Eynden, G., Baehner, F. L., Penault-Llorca, F., Perez, E. A., Thompson, E. A., Symmans, W. F., Richardson, A. L., Brock, J., Criscitiello, C., Bailey, H., Ignatiadis, M., FLORIS, G., Sparano, J., Kos, Z., Nielsen, T., Rimm, D. L., Allison, K. H., Reis-Filho, J. S., Loibl, S., Sotiriou, C., Viale, G., Badve, S., Adams, S., Willard-Gallo, K., Loi, S., & INTERNATIONAL, T. W. G. (2015). The evaluation of tumor-infiltrating lymphocytes (TILs) in breast cancer: Recommendations by an International TILs working group 2014. *Annals of Oncology, 26*, 259–271.

Schellens, J. H. M., Marabelle, A., Zeigenfuss, S., Ding, J., Pruitt, S. K., & Chung, H. C. (2017). Pembrolizumab for previously treated advanced cervical squamous cell cancer: Preliminary results from the phase 2 KEYNOTE-158 studye. *Journal of Clinical Oncology, 35*(15_suppl), 5514.

Segal, N. H., Parsons, D. W., Peggs, K. S., Velculescu, V., Kinzler, K. W., Vogelstein, B., & Allison, J. P. (2008). Epitope landscape in breast and colorectal cancer. *Cancer Research, 68*, 889–892.

Segal, N. H., Antonia, S. J., Brahmer, J. R., Maio, M., Blake-Haskins, A., Li, X., Vasselli, J., Ibrahim, R. A., Lutzky, J., & Khieif, S. (2014). Preliminary data from a multi-arm expansion study of MEDI4736, an anti-PD-L1 antibody. *Journal of Clinical Oncology, 32*(15_suppl), 3002.

Segal, N. H., Ou, S. H. I., Balmanoukian, A. S., Massarelli, E., Brahmer, J. R., Weiss, J., Schoffski, P., Antonia, S. J., Massard, C., Zandberg, D. P., Maher, C., Khleif, S., Jin, X., Rebelatto, M., Steele, K., Antal, J., Gupta, A., & Spreafico, A. (2016). Updated safety and efficacy of durvalumab (MEDI4736), an anti-PD-L 1 antibody, in patients from a squamous cell carcinoma of the head and neck (SCCHN) expansion cohort. *Annals of Oncology, 27*.

Topalian, S. L., Hodi, F. S., Brahmer, J. R., Gettinger, S. N., Smith, D. C., Mcdermott, D. F., Powderly, J. D., Carvajal, R. D., Sosman, J. A., Atkins, M. B., Leming, P. D., Spigel, D. R., Antonia, S. J., Horn, L., Drake, C. G., Pardoll, D. M., Chen, L., Sharfman, W. H., Anders, R. A., Taube, J. M., Mcmiller, T. L., Xu, H., Korman, A. J., Jure-Kunkel, M., Agrawal, S., Mcdonald, D., Kollia, G. D., Gupta, A., Wigginton, J. M., & Sznol, M. (2012). Safety, activity, and immune correlates of anti-PD-1 antibody in cancer. *The New England Journal of Medicine, 366*, 2443–2454.

Varga, A., Piha-Paul, S. A., Ott, P. A., Mehnert, J. M., Berton-Rigaud, D., Johnson, E. A., Cheng, J. D., Yuan, S., Rubin, E. H., & Matei, D. E. (2015). Antitumor activity and safety of pembrolizumab in patients (pts) with PD-L1 positive advanced ovarian cancer: Interim results from a phase Ib study. *Journal of Clinical Oncology, 33*(15_suppl), 5510.

Wang, B. J., Bao, J. J., Wang, J. Z., Wang, Y., Jiang, M., Xing, M. Y., Zhang, W. G., Qi, J. Y., Roggendorf, M., Lu, M. J., & Yang, D. L. (2011). Immunostaining of PD-1/PD-Ls in liver tissues of patients with hepatitis and hepatocellular carcinoma. *World Journal of Gastroenterology, 17*, 3322–3329.

Weber, J. S., D'angelo, S. P., Minor, D., Hodi, F. S., Gutzmer, R., Neyns, B., Hoeller, C., Khushalani, N. I., Miller, W. H., Lao, C. D., Linette, G. P., Thomas, L., Lorigan, P., Grossmann, K. F., Hassel, J. C., Maio, M., Sznol, M., Ascierto, P. A., Mohr, P., Chmielowski, B., Bryce, A., Svane, I. M., Grob, J. J., Krackhardt, A. M., Horak, C., Lambert, A., Yang, A. S., & Larkin, J. (2015). Nivolumab versus chemotherapy in patients with advanced melanoma who progressed after anti-CTLA-4 treatment (CheckMate 037): A randomised, controlled, open-label, phase 3 trial. *The Lancet Oncology, 16*, 375–384.

Zhang, M. H., Dong, Y. D., Liu, H. T., Wang, Y., Zhao, S., Xuan, Q. J., Wang, Y., & Zhang, Q. Y. (2016). The clinicopathological and prognostic significance of PD-L1 expression in gastric cancer: A meta-analysis of 10 studies with 1,901 patients. *Scientific Reports, 94*(6), e515.

Chapter 9
Management of Immune-Related Adverse Events from Immune Checkpoint Inhibitor Therapy

Lisa Kottschade

Contents

Introduction

The landscape of cancer therapy has changed dramatically over the last decade. From traditional cytotoxic chemotherapy, small-molecule inhibitors, to the explosion of immune checkpoint inhibitor (ICI) therapy, the paradigm of cancer therapy will never be the same. Unfortunately, with these advances comes additional toxicity and morbidity. The side-effect profile for ICI therapy is distinctly different from that of chemotherapy and/or small-molecule therapy, in that toxicity is directly related to over-activation of the immune system. Additionally, whereas side effects from chemotherapy and small-molecule therapy will usually resolve on their own after withdrawal of the agent, toxicity from ICI therapy can have delayed onset and last for months after drug withdrawal. Therefore, early recognition and intervention are imperative for patients on ICI therapy to prevent morbidity and mortality.

L. Kottschade (✉)
Medical Oncology, Mayo Clinic, Rochester, MN, USA

© Springer International Publishing AG 2018
H. Dong, S.N. Markovic (eds.), *The Basics of Cancer Immunotherapy*,
https://doi.org/10.1007/978-3-319-70622-1_9

While the three main classes of ICI therapy (anti-CTLA-4, anti-PD-1, and anti-PD-L1 inhibitors) exert their effects on different targets of the immune system, their side-effect profile is similar and overlapping, and thus treatment for immune-related adverse events (irAEs) is somewhat universal across drug classes. irAEs are usually classified by organ system; however, treatment (with a few exceptions) is a balancing act designed at dampening the immune response to reverse the particular side effect, without losing the efficacy against the tumor.

The most common organ classes involved with irAE's are gastrointestinal, dermatological, and endocrine systems. Less common, but often times more serious, are those of the pulmonary, neurologic, hematologic, and cardiac systems.

Gastrointestinal

Immune related adverse events (irAE's) of a gastrointestinal etiology usually manifest in the forms of diarrhea, colitis, and/or autoimmune hepatotoxicity (Beck et al. 2006; Bertrand et al. 2015; Eigentler et al. 2016; Hodi et al. 2014; Huffman et al. 2017; Kim et al. 2013; Kottschade et al., 2016). Diarrhea/colitis is most commonly seen with anti-CTLA-4 therapy both as single therapy and in combination with anti-PD-1 therapy (Hodi et al. 2010; Postow et al. 2015; Robert et al. 2011, 2015a, b; Wolchok et al. 2013). Incidence rates vary from 30% (any grade) with single-agent anti-CTLA-4 therapy to approximately 50% (any grade) for combination anti-CTLA-4/anti-PD-1 therapy (Hodi et al., 2010; Postow et al. 2015; Robert et al. 2011, 2015a, b; Wolchok et al. 2013). Of note, gastrointestinal side effects of this nature are far less common with anti-PD-1 therapy alone, where < 20% of patients experience diarrhea/colitis (Robert et al. 2015a, b; Co 2014). Symptoms can present as simply as a mild increase in the number of stools to profuse diarrhea that can lead to dehydration and require hospitalization. Rarely, fatal bowel perforations have been documented, emphasizing the necessity to recognize and treat early signs of intestinal toxicity (Larkin et al. 2015; Eggermont et al. 2015). Careful assessment of the patient's bowel habits is crucial for early detection and intervention. Patients should be assessed both for the number of stools and consistency. Red flags would include hematochezia, mucous in the stool, fever, abdominal pain, and/or signs of dehydration (hypotension, weakness). Most patients with grade 1 diarrhea (an increase of fewer than four stools per 24 hours), can be managed with conservative methods (Kottschade et al. 2016). These would include bland diet (BRAT diet), increase of fluids, and close monitoring for any increase in the number of stools. Antidiarrheal agents can be used with caution, but generally should be avoided, as these can mask worsening of symptoms and have no overall impact on any underlying colitis. Treatment can usually be continued cautiously in patients with grade 1 diarrhea. Patients with > grade 2 diarrhea will need intervention, usually with steroids to prevent further worsening of symptoms. Treatment should be held for those with grade 2 diarrhea until symptoms return to ≤ grade 1 and steroid dosing is 10 mg or less of prednisone (or equivalent). Those with grade 3 or higher diarrhea will likely need to discontinue treatment, with the following exception: As anti-CTLA-4 agents generally have higher rates of diarrhea, patients who have recovered to < grade 2 and have discontinued steroids can be re-challenged with single-agent anti-PD-1, including those who developed diarrhea on dual checkpoint inhibitor blockade. For patients with grade 3 or higher diarrhea, or those that are steroid refractory at any grade, they should be evaluated by a gastroenterologist and have an evaluation by flexible sigmoidoscopy and/or colonoscopy to assess the extent of colitis as well as assess need for biologic modifiers to manage the diarrhea (Kottschade et al. 2016).

Hepatotoxicity is a direct result of the inflammation of hepatocytes in the liver from T-cell infiltration (Weber et al. 2013). Left untreated, autoimmune hepatitis can lead to liver failure and eventual death. Often patients present with asymptomatic transaminitis and/or hyperbilirubinemia detected on routine liver function tests (LFTs) (Weber et al. 2013). Patients should be assessed prior to each infusion of ICI therapy on the following laboratory values: AST, ALT, alkaline phosphatase, and total and direct bilirubin. Additionally, patients presenting with abdominal pain, profound fatigue and/or jaundice should also be urgently evaluated for autoimmune hepatitis. All patients should be ruled out for other causes of symptoms, especially progressive hepatic metastasis. Management includes the following: Grade 1—careful monitoring of LFTs weekly in-between ICI therapy dosing. Grade 2 and above—ICI therapy should be held, with initiation of steroids. LFTs should be monitored twice weekly until ≤ grade 1. Once LFTs have stabilized and/or started decreasing, steroids can be slowly tapered with continued frequent monitoring of LFTs. Re-challenge of ICI therapy can be done cautiously, with careful LFT monitoring as autoimmune hepatitis can re-appear. Patients with grade 3 or higher and/or autoimmune hepatitis that is refractory to steroids should be referred to a hepatologist for further management (Huffman et al. 2017).

Dermatological

The most common irAE with ICI therapy is that of skin toxicity. Patients will typically present with a maculo-papular rash, mimicking that of a drug reaction, often times with significant pruritus (Hodi et al. 2003). It should be noted that patients can present with pruritus only with no visible skin lesions. Rashes are more common with anti-CTLA-4 based therapy (~ 40% with monotherapy and up to 70% with dual ICI therapy), single-agent anti-PD-1 or PD-L1 therapy has a lower incidence rate of approximately 25% (Postow et al. 2015; Wolchok et al. 2013; Ibrahim et al. 2011; Weber et al. 2012). Grading and therefore subsequent treatment for dermatologic irAEs is usually based on amount of body surface area (BSA) involved with lesions. Patients with grade 1 (< 20% BSA involvement) can usually be managed conservatively with antihistamines and topical corticosteroids. Treatment with ICI therapy can continue cautiously, as long as there is no worsening of symptoms and/or significant increase in the lesions. For patients experiencing grade 2 rash

(20–50% BSA involvement), treatment should include the addition of low-dose steroids (~ 0.5–1 mg/kg of prednisone or equivalent), and ICI treatment should be withheld until improvement to ≤ grade 1 and steroid dosing has been tapered to 10 mg of prednisone or equivalent. While rash may clear rapidly with the introduction of oral steroids, providers should be cautioned that a rapid taper of steroids can cause an acute rebound of the rash. Patients with grade 3 (> 50% BSA involvement) or higher rash, and/or rash refractory to steroids should be initiated on higher doses of steroids, with referral to a dermatologist for additional management. Treatment with ICI therapy should generally be discontinued in patients with grade 3 or higher dermatological toxicity. Patients with blister-like lesions, fever, or lesions in the oral mucosa or genital region should be evaluated urgently to rule out more serious conditions including Steven's Johnson Syndrome or toxic epidermal necrolysis.

Endocrine Toxicity

irAEs of the endocrine system are usually classified into two categories, those that involve the thyroid and those that involve the pituitary-gonadal-adrenal (PGA) axis (Bertrand et al. 2015; Larkin et al. 2015; Gonzalez-Rodriguez & Rodriguez-Abreu 2016). Diagnosis of disorders of the endocrine system can be difficult to sort out, as many will present with generalized constitutional symptoms (fatigue, mild headache, etc.), and therefore this class of irAEs is often misdiagnosed. Additionally patients may be on steroids for other irAEs and consequently endocrine-related irAEs are often masked during this time and only become obvious during steroid tapers (i.e., secondary adrenal insufficiency), and thus their etiology (i.e., irAE vs. prolonged steroid use) is almost impossible to discern (Beck et al. 2006; Ryder et al. 2014).

Thyroid dysfunction can present in two forms, hyperthyroidism and hypothyroidism. The most common scenario is patients presenting with asymptomatic suppression of TSH, and high free T4 and/or T3 on routine thyroid function monitoring. Some patients will have transient tachycardia associated with this that will require temporary low-dose beta blockade. Often this phase of thyroiditis will resolve on its own to euthyroid levels within 4–6 weeks and will not require further intervention (Kottschade et al. 2016; Ryder et al. 2014). However, there is a group of patients that will progress and develop overt hypothyroidism (defined as a TSH > 10). Patients who progress to overt hypothyroidism and/or present with symptomatic hypothyroidism should be started on thyroid replacement therapy (Kottschade et al. 2016; Ryder et al. 2014). Usual starting replacement doses for levothyroxine are 1.6 μg/kg body weight; however, patients who are asymptomatic and/or have pre-existing cardiac conditions can be started at slightly lower doses. Patients should continue to have their thyroid function checked every 3–6 weeks while on ICI therapy, with dose adjustments of levothyroxine as necessary to keep TSH within the normal reference range of around 0.5–4 (Kottschade et al. 2016; Ryder et al. 2014). Patients with isolated autoimmune thyroiditis can continue to receive ICI therapy, with little to no interruption in treatment cycles.

Dysfunction of the PGA axis most commonly manifests as hypophysitis (Ryder et al. 2014; Corsello et al. 2013). Hypophysitis usually will present with acute severe headache, nausea, possible vomiting, and often profound fatigue. Given the similarity of these symptoms to acute intracranial metastatic disease, this should always be in the differential diagnosis. The diagnosis of hypophysitis is usually made based on low to undetectable morning cortisol and low ACTH (adrenocotico-tropic hormone) levels (Corsello et al. 2013). Magnetic resonance imaging (MRI) is recommended in these situations to rule out intracranial disease and other neuro-logical irAEs (i.e., encephalitis), and can also assist in the diagnosis of pituitary dysfunction; however, specific views of the pituitary gland should be requested dur-ing the MRI as often these are not routinely done as part of a regular MRI exam. It should be noted that during the acute phase of hypophysitis approximately 75% of patients will have enhancement/enlargement of the pituitary gland on MRI imaging (Corsello et al. 2013). Treatment of this irAE centers around decreasing inflamma-tion in the pituitary gland and thus relieving associated symptoms. Most patients will require at least 1 mg/kg of prednisone (or equivalent) for relief, but some with severe symptoms will require up to 2 mg/kg initially and may require hospitaliza-tion (Kottschade et al. 2016). However, distinct from other irAEs, high-dose ste-roids can relieve the acute symptoms of hypophysitis in 1–2 weeks, and thereafter steroids can be more rapidly tapered to physiologic replacement levels (provided other irAEs are not present) (Kottschade et al. 2016). Unfortunately, most of these patients are left with permanent secondary adrenal insufficiency and require lifeline glucocorticoid replacement. Of note, ICI therapy should be held during the acute phase; however, once patients are asymptomatic and have tapered to lower doses of prednisone without recurrence of symptoms, ICI therapy may be safely resumed. While rare, primary adrenal insufficiency (adrenal crisis) has been seen with these agents (Hodi et al. 2010; Corsello et al. 2013; Brahmer et al. 2012; Hamid et al. 2013). This is a life-threatening emergency that needs to be recognized and treated immediately to prevent increased morbidity and mortality. Patients should have ICI therapy withheld until they are asymptomatic, electrolytes are normal, and steroids have been tapered.

Pulmonary Toxicity

While a much less common irAE, pulmonary toxicity can develop and progress swiftly, leading to significant morbidity and even death. Pulmonary toxicity or pneumonitis (as it usually presents) can often start subtly, with a minor cough and slight dyspnea on exertion, and rapidly progress to hypoxemia with significant respiratory compromise (Postow et al. 2015; Wolchok et al. 2013; Larkin et al. 2015). This irAE tends to be commonly incorrectly and undertreated of the immune-related events, as presenting symptoms are often mistaken and assumed to be from bacterial pneumonia. Standard plain chest radiography usually will reveal minor changes and/or small consolidations that are labeled as "pneumonia." Patients are subsequently inappropriately placed on antibiotics and often continued on ICI treatment. The actual incidence of pneumonitis seems to vary amongst the malignancies as well as treatment regimens (Hodi et al. 2010, 2014; Postow et al. 2015; Robert et al. 2015a, b; Wolchok et al. 2013; Larkin et al. 2015; Hamid et al., 2013; Ribas et al. 2013; Sznol et al. 2017; Topalian et al. 2012). In single-agent anti-PD-1 therapy, agents tend to have a higher incidence over anti-CTLA-4 agents alone (Hodi et al. 2010; Postow et al. 2015; Robert et al. 2015a, b; Wolchok et al. 2013; Larkin et al. 2015; Sznol et al. 2017). However, combination ICI therapy tends to have an even higher incidence rate, and in addition there seems to be a higher rate amongst those with primary lung cancer and/or patients with previous pulmonary radiation (Postow et al. 2015; Wolchok et al. 2013; Sznol et al. 2017; Brahmer et al. 2015). For patients with suspected pulmonary irAE, workup should include the following: comprehensive pulmonary history (to assess for pre-existing conditions that may complicate the diagnostic picture), pulse oximetry, cross-section radiographic images of the chest (i.e., CT scans), pulmonary function testing as indicated, and consideration of bronchoscopy to rule out infectious etiology (Kottschade et al. 2016). It should be noted, however, that in cases where radiographic infiltrates/interstitial inflammation is noted, especially in patients who are symptomatic, steroids should not be withheld in patients while awaiting infectious workup, due to the serious nature and usual rapid decline these patients can experience if left untreated (Kottschade et al. 2016). For patients who have grade 1 toxicity (radiographic findings only), these patients can generally be continued on therapy with careful monitoring, which may include more frequent cross-section imaging of the chest. Patients with grade 2 or higher toxicity should have treatment withheld (grade 3 or 4 should discontinue therapy) and should be started on systemic steroids. Patients should be monitored closely for any worsening of respiratory status and hypoxia. Patients with abnormal oxygen saturation should be hospitalized and receive high-dose IV steroids (solumedrol 500–1,000 mg daily) until respiratory status improves (Kottschade et al. 2016). Patients who are steroid refractory or do not improve quickly with steroids should undergo a bronchoscopy, for further diagnostic inquiry (Kottschade et al. 2016). Patients with grade 2 toxicity can be rechallenged with ICI therapy once steroids have been tapered to 10 mg of prednisone daily. Those with grade 3 or 4 toxicity should not receive further ICI therapy, due to the risk of further respiratory compromise.

Renal Toxicity

Rarely patients can develop renal toxicity while on ICI therapy, usually manifesting in the form of acute interstitial nephritis. Incidence rates for renal toxicity are relatively low, ranging from around 1% in single-agent PD-1 trials to approximately 3–4% in patients undergoing therapy with dual checkpoint inhibitor therapy (anti-PD-1 and anti-CTLA-4) (Fadel et al. 2009; Izzedine et al. 2014; Voskens et al. 2013). Routine monitoring would include serum creatinine at baseline and prior to each dose of ICI therapy. Increases in creatinine levels can be an early indicator of impending renal toxicity and should be monitored more closely. Patients with mild elevations (grade 1) can usually continue ICI treatment with more frequent monitoring (i.e., weekly creatinine levels). Patients with grade 2 or higher irAEs should have treatment withheld and be referred to a nephrologist for further workup and consideration of renal biopsy to rule out acute interstitial nephritis. Patients should be started on steroids to prevent further renal damage (grade 2: 0.5 mg/kg of prednisone, grade 3 or 4 irAE: 1–2 mg/kg of prednisone). Those with grade 2 or less toxicity can be re-challenged with further ICI therapy, with close observation.

Neurological Toxicity

While rare (~1%), neurological toxicity can be severe and life-threatening. These toxicities can present late, even after ICI therapy has been discontinued. Neurological toxicity can range from peripheral neuropathy or neuritis to encephalitis and Guillain-Barre syndrome (acute inflammatory demyelinating polyneuropathy, AIDP) (Sznol et al. 2017; Bompaire et al. 2012; Bot et al. 2013; Hunter et al. 2009; Johnson et al. 2013; Wilgenhof & Neyns 2011). Many of these side effects can mimic side effects from CNS metastasis, meaning this possibility must be immediately ruled out, and once done strong consideration must be given to neurological side effects from ICI therapy, which require urgent intervention to prevent significant morbidity and/or mortality. Treatment of neurologic irAEs is dependent on the type and severity of irAE and should be done in collaboration with a neurologist. Patients experiencing grade 1 peripheral neuropathy (PN) should be closely observed, and those who have grade 2 PN should have treatment withheld. Therapy should be permanently discontinued for patients with grade 3 or 4 PN. Patients who experience more significant neurological toxicity (i.e., AIDP) should have ICI therapy Immune-related adverse events (irAE's):neurological toxicity permanently discontinued.

Ocular Toxicity

Uveitis, episcleritis, iritis, conjunctivitis, and orbital inflammation have been reported in the literature with ICI therapy, with the least common being uveitis (Brahmer et al. 2012; Abdel-Rahman et al., 2017; Robinson et al. 2004; Wolchok et al. 2010). All patients who report any sort of ocular symptoms (i.e., pain in the eye, light intolerance, or visual changes) should be immediately referred to an ophthalmologist for appropriate workup and treatment. For those patients who are only experiencing mild dry eyes in the absence of other symptoms (i.e., pain), it is recommended that they start lubricating eye drops, and counselled to immediately report any changes in symptoms. Those with more serious ocular toxicity may require topical steroid drops and/or intraocular injections. Rarely, patients will require treatment with oral steroids.

Rheumatological Toxicity

There have been recent case reports in the literature of patients on ICI therapy who have experienced side effects that mimic rheumatological-type syndromes. Those that have been described include dry mouth and eyes (sicca-like syndrome), inflammatory arthritis, and psoriasis (Sznol et al. 2017; Fadel et al. 2009). Given the relatively rare nature of these syndromes, patients should be referred to a rheumatologist for further investigation and management. While some patients with mild symptoms can be managed and continue on ICI therapy cautiously, others will require discontinuation and intervention with steroids or other immune modulators.

Conclusion

While immune checkpoint inhibitors have provided new hope to patients with cancer, the side-effect profile associated with this class of agents is unlike anything that has been experienced in oncology so far. irAEs are unique in that they develop as a direct result of manipulation and stimulation of the immune system, thus their management is different to those with chemotherapy and/or small-molecule inhibitors. Unlike side effects experienced with other oncologic agents, irAEs do not usually resolve with simple withdrawal or dose modification, and require intervention with steroids or other agents to dampen the immune response. With the rapid expansion of ICI therapy in both solid tumors and hematologic malignancies, early recognition and appropriate management by providers to prevent long-term morbidity is essential.

References

Abdel-Rahman, O., Oweira, H., Petrausch, U., Helbling, D., Schmidt, J., Mannhart, M., et al. (2017). Immune-related ocular toxicities in solid tumor patients treated with immune checkpoint inhibitors: A systematic review. *Expert Review of Anticancer Therapy, 17*(4), 387–394.

Beck, K. E., Blansfield, J. A., Tran, K. Q., Feldman, A. L., Hughes, M. S., Royal, R. E., et al. (2006). Enterocolitis in patients with cancer after antibody blockade of cytotoxic T-lymphocyte-associated antigen 4. *Journal of Clinical Oncology, 24*(15), 2283–2289.

Bertrand, A., Kostine, M., Barnetche, T., Truchetet, M. E., & Schaeverbeke, T. (2015). Immune related adverse events associated with anti-CTLA-4 antibodies: Systematic review and meta-analysis. *BMC Medicine, 13*, 211.

Bompaire, F., Mateus, C., Taillia, H., De Greslan, T., Lahutte, M., Sallansonnet-Froment, M., et al. (2012). Severe meningo-radiculo-neuritis associated with ipilimumab. *Investigational New Drugs, 30*(6), 2407–2410. https://doi.org/10.1007/s10637-011-9787-1. Epub 2012 Jan 11.

Bot, I., Blank, C. U., Boogerd, W., & Brandsma, D. (2013). Neurological immune-related adverse events of ipilimumab. *Practical Neurology, 13*(4), 278–280. https://doi.org/10.1136/practneurol-2012-000447. Epub 2013 Mar 13.

Brahmer, J. R., Tykodi, S. S., Chow, L. Q., Hwu, W. J., Topalian, S. L., Hwu, P., et al. (2012). Safety and activity of anti-PD-L1 antibody in patients with advanced cancer. *The New England Journal of Medicine, 366*(26), 2455–2465. https://doi.org/10.1056/NEJMoa1200694. Epub 2012 Jun 2.

Brahmer, J., Reckamp, K. L., Baas, P., Crino, L., Eberhardt, W. E., Poddubskaya, E., et al. (2015). Nivolumab versus docetaxel in advanced squamous-cell non-small-cell lung cancer. *The New England Journal of Medicine, 373*(2), 123–135.

Co, M. (2014). Keytruda (pembrolizumab) for injection: Highlights of prescribing information. Accessed 19 April 2015 at http://www.merck.com/product/usa/pi_circulars/k/keytruda/keytruda_pi.pdf.

Corsello, S. M., Barnabei, A., Marchetti, P., De Vecchis, L., Salvatori, R., & Torino, F. (2013). Endocrine side effects induced by immune checkpoint inhibitors. *The Journal of Clinical Endocrinology and Metabolism, 98*(4), 1361–1375. https://doi.org/10.1210/jc.2012-4075. Epub 2013 Mar 7.

Eggermont, A. M., Chiarion-Sileni, V., Grob, J. J., Dummer, R., Wolchok, J. D., Schmidt, H., et al. (2015). Adjuvant ipilimumab versus placebo after complete resection of high-risk stage III melanoma (EORTC 18071): A randomised, double-blind, phase 3 trial. *The Lancet Oncology, 16*(5), 522–530.

Eigentler, T. K., Hassel, J. C., Berking, C., Aberle, J., Bachmann, O., Grunwald, V., et al. (2016). Diagnosis, monitoring and management of immune-related adverse drug reactions of anti-PD-1 antibody therapy. *Cancer Treatment Reviews, 45*, 7–18.

Fadel, F., El Karoui, K., & Knebelmann, B. (2009). Anti-CTLA4 antibody-induced lupus nephritis. *The New England Journal of Medicine, 361*(2), 211–212. https://doi.org/10.1056/NEJMc0904283.

Gonzalez-Rodriguez, E., Rodriguez-Abreu, D., & Spanish Group for Cancer I-B. (2016). Immune checkpoint inhibitors: Review and management of endocrine adverse events. *The Oncologist, 21*(7), 804–816.

Hamid, O., Robert, C., Daud, A., Hodi, F. S., Hwu, W. J., Kefford, R., et al. (2013). Safety and tumor responses with lambrolizumab (anti-PD-1) in melanoma. *The New England Journal of Medicine, 369*(2), 134–144.

Hodi, F. S., Mihm, M. C., Soiffer, R. J., Haluska, F. G., Butler, M., Seiden, M. V., et al. (2003). Biologic activity of cytotoxic T lymphocyte-associated antigen 4 antibody blockade in previously vaccinated metastatic melanoma and ovarian carcinoma patients. *Proceedings of the National Academy of Sciences of the United States of America, 100*(8), 4712–4717. Epub 2003 Apr 7.

Hodi, F. S., O'Day, S. J., McDermott, D. F., Weber, R. W., Sosman, J. A., Haanen, J. B., et al. (2010). Improved survival with ipilimumab in patients with metastatic melanoma. *The New England Journal of Medicine, 363*(8), 711–723. https://doi.org/10.1056/NEJMoa1003466. Epub 2010 Jun 5.

Hodi, F. S., Lee, S., McDermott, D. F., Rao, U. N., Butterfield, L. H., Tarhini, A. A., et al. (2014). Ipilimumab plus sargramostim vs ipilimumab alone for treatment of metastatic melanoma: A randomized clinical trial. *JAMA, 312*(17), 1744–1753.

Huffman, B. M., Kottschade, L. A., Kamath, P. S., & Markovic, S. N. (2017). Hepatotoxicity after immune checkpoint inhibitor therapy in melanoma: Natural progression and management. *American Journal of Clinical Oncology, 2*(2), 204–210.

Hunter, G., Voll, C., & Robinson, C. A. (2009). Autoimmune inflammatory myopathy after treatment with ipilimumab. *The Canadian Journal of Neurological Sciences, 36*(4), 518–520.

Ibrahim, R. A., Berman, D. M., DePril, V., Humphrey, R. W., Chen, T., Messina, M., et al. (2011). Ipilimumab safety profile: Summary of findings from completed trials in advanced melanoma 2011. *Journal of Clinical Oncology, 118*(1), 109–116.

Izzedine, H., Gueutin, V., Gharbi, C., Mateus, C., Robert, C., Routier, E., et al. (2014). Kidney injuries related to ipilimumab. *Investigational New Drugs, 32*(4), 769–773. https://doi.org/10.1007/s10637-014-0092-7. Epub 2014 Apr 1.

Johnson, D. B., Wallender, E. K., Cohen, D. N., Likhari, S. S., Zwerner, J. P., Powers, J. G., et al. (2013). Severe cutaneous and neurologic toxicity in melanoma patients during vemurafenib administration following anti-PD-1 therapy. *Cancer Immunology Research, 1*(6), 373–377. https://doi.org/10.1158/2326-6066.CIR-13-0092.

Kim, K. W., Ramaiya, N. H., Krajewski, K. M., Jagannathan, J. P., Tirumani, S. H., Srivastava, A., et al. (2013). Ipilimumab associated hepatitis: Imaging and clinicopathologic findings. *Investigational New Drugs, 31*(4), 1071–1077. https://doi.org/10.1007/s10637-013-9939-6. Epub 2013 Feb 14.

Kottschade, L., Brys, A., Peikert, T., Ryder, M., Raffals, L., Brewer, J., et al. (2016). A multidisciplinary approach to toxicity management of modern immune checkpoint inhibitors in cancer therapy. *Melanoma Research, 26*(5), 469–480.

Larkin, J., Chiarion-Sileni, V., Gonzalez, R., Grob, J. J., Cowey, C. L., Lao, C. D., et al. (2015). Combined nivolumab and ipilimumab or monotherapy in untreated melanoma. *The New England Journal of Medicine, 373*(1), 23–34.

Postow, M. A., Chesney, J., Pavlick, A. C., Robert, C., Grossmann, K., McDermott, D., et al. (2015). Nivolumab and ipilimumab versus ipilimumab in untreated melanoma. *The New England Journal of Medicine, 372*(21), 2006–2017.

Ribas, A., Kefford, R., Marshall, M. A., Punt, C. J., Haanen, J. B., Marmol, M., et al. (2013). Phase III randomized clinical trial comparing tremelimumab with standard-of-care chemotherapy in patients with advanced melanoma. *Journal of Clinical Oncology, 31*(5), 616–622.

Robert, C., Thomas, L., Bondarenko, I., O'Day, S., Weber, J., Garbe, C., et al. (2011). Ipilimumab plus dacarbazine for previously untreated metastatic melanoma. *The New England Journal of Medicine, 364*(26), 2517–2526. https://doi.org/10.1056/NEJMoa1104621. Epub 2011 Jun 5.

Robert, C., Long, G. V., Brady, B., Dutriaux, C., Maio, M., Mortier, L., et al. (2015a). Nivolumab in previously untreated melanoma without BRAF mutation. *The New England Journal of Medicine, 372*(4), 320–330. https://doi.org/10.1056/NEJMoa1412082. Epub 2014 Nov 16.

Robert, C., Schachter, J., Long, G. V., Arance, A., Grob, J. J., Mortier, L., et al. (2015b). Pembrolizumab versus ipilimumab in advanced melanoma. *The New England Journal of Medicine, 372*(26), 2521–2532.

Robinson, M. R., Chan, C. C., Yang, J. C., Rubin, B. I., Gracia, G. J., Sen, H. N., et al. (2004). Cytotoxic T lymphocyte-associated antigen 4 blockade in patients with metastatic melanoma: A new cause of uveitis. *Journal of Immunotherapy, 27*(6), 478–479.

Ryder, M., Callahan, M., Postow, M. A., Wolchok, J., & Fagin, J. A. (2014). Endocrine-related adverse events following ipilimumab in patients with advanced melanoma: A comprehensive retrospective review from a single institution. *Endocrine-Related Cancer, 21*(2), 371–381.

Sznol, M., Ferrucci, P. F., Hogg, D., Atkins, M. B., Wolter, P., Guidoboni, M., et al. (2017). Pooled analysis safety profile of nivolumab and ipilimumab combination therapy in patients with advanced melanoma. *Journal of Clinical Oncology*, JCO2016721167.

Topalian, S. L., Hodi, F. S., Brahmer, J. R., Gettinger, S. N., Smith, D. C., McDermott, D. F., et al. (2012). Safety, activity, and immune correlates of anti-PD-1 antibody in cancer. *The New England Journal of Medicine, 366*(26), 2443–2554. https://doi.org/10.1056/NEJMoa1200690. Epub 2012 Jun 2.

Voskens, C. J., Goldinger, S. M., Loquai, C., Robert, C., Kaehler, K. C., Berking, C., et al. (2013). The price of tumor control: An analysis of rare side effects of anti-CTLA-4 therapy in metastatic melanoma from the ipilimumab network. *PLoS One, 8*(1), e53745. https://doi.org/10.1371/journal.pone.0053745. Epub 2013 Jan 14.

Weber, J. S., Kahler, K. C., & Hauschild, A. (2012). Management of immune-related adverse events and kinetics of response with ipilimumab. *Journal of Clinical Oncology, 30*(21), 2691–2697. https://doi.org/10.1200/JCO.2012.41.6750. Epub 2012 May 21.

Weber, J. S., Dummer, R., de Pril, V., Lebbe, C., & Hodi, F. S. (2013). Patterns of onset and resolution of immune-related adverse events of special interest with ipilimumab: Detailed safety analysis from a phase 3 trial in patients with advanced melanoma. *Cancer, 119*(9), 1675–1682. https://doi.org/10.1002/cncr.27969. Epub 2013 Feb 7.

Wilgenhof, S., & Neyns, B. (2011). Anti-CTLA-4 antibody-induced Guillain-Barre syndrome in a melanoma patient. *Annals of Oncology, 22*(4), 991–993. https://doi.org/10.1093/annonc/mdr028. Epub 2011 Feb 28.

Wolchok, J. D., Neyns, B., Linette, G., Negrier, S., Lutzky, J., Thomas, L., et al. (2010). Ipilimumab monotherapy in patients with pretreated advanced melanoma: A randomised, double-blind, multicentre, phase 2, dose-ranging study. *The Lancet Oncology, 11*(2), 155–164. https://doi.org/10.1016/S470-2045(09)70334-1. Epub 2009 Dec 8.

Wolchok, J. D., Kluger, H., Callahan, M. K., Postow, M. A., Rizvi, N. A., Lesokhin, A. M., et al. (2013). Nivolumab plus ipilimumab in advanced melanoma. *The New England Journal of Medicine, 369*(2), 122–133. https://doi.org/10.1056/NEJMoa1302369. Epub 2013 Jun 2.

Chapter 10
Resources for Patients

Immunotherapy is rapidly changing the ways how we treat cancer and is bringing hope to cancer patients. New medications and novel treatment modalities are constantly evolving, thanks to the ongoing research efforts. Given the rapid advances in this field, we strongly encourage our patients to discuss treatment options with their providers to formulate an individualized treatment plan, including potential participation in ongoing clinical trials.

Cancer immunotherapy has a unique side-effect profile compared to other conventional cancer therapies, such as chemotherapy. In addition to patient education prior to the initiation of treatment, it is very important for patients to inform their oncologic providers of the onset of side effects or any new symptoms, because early recognition and treatment of immunotherapy-related side effects is critical, and self-medicating for common symptoms (e.g., diarrhea) is strongly discouraged.

We understand the scope of this book does not allow for the discussion of all the details regarding cancer immunotherapy; therefore, we refer patients to the following links for further information. However, an open and ongoing communication with your provider, instead of the overwhelming amount of information on the internet, is always the most effective way to address questions related to your treatment.

Clinical trial information:

www.Clinicaltrials.gov

American cancer society:

https://www.cancer.org/treatment/treatments-and-side-effects/treatment-types/immunotherapy.html

Micromedex (information about drug facts, including side effects):

http://www.micromedexsolutions.com

Y. Yan (✉)
Division of Medical Oncology, Mayo Clinic, Rochester, MN, USA

© Springer International Publishing AG 2018
H. Dong, S.N. Markovic (eds.), *The Basics of Cancer Immunotherapy*,
https://doi.org/10.1007/978-3-319-70622-1_10

Lymphoma research foundation:
www.lymphoma.org
Leukemia & Lymphoma Society:
www.lls.org
American Society of Hematology:
http://www.hematology.org/Patients/

Index